Table of Contents

Charting

Regulatory Compliance

Reporting

Case Studies

Certified Electronic Health Record Specialist (CEHRS)
Study Guide

Contributors

Rebecca Harmon, MPM, RHIA
Contributing Writer

Mandy Tallmadge, BS Communication
Product Developer

Nicole Burke, BS Journalism
Product Developer

Nicole Hicks, BA Film & Video
Media Developer

INTELLECTUAL PROPERTY NOTICE

IMPORTANT NOTICE TO THE READER

solely at your own risk. Health care professionals need to use their own clinical judgment in interpreting the content of this publication, and details such as medications, dosages, and laboratory tests and results should always be confirmed with other resources.

This publication may contain health- or medical-related materials that are sexually explicit. If you find these materials offensive, you may not want to use this publication.

>> INTRODUCTION

Learning Objectives

After reading this study guide, you will be able to:

- *Explain the duties and responsibilities of an EHR specialist.*

- *Effectively use EHR certified software and integrated equipment.*

- *Describe how you are involved with a facility's insurance and billing process, including generating reports and statements.*

- *Monitor charts for completeness and accuracy in documentation.*

- *Execute file maintenance procedures.*

- *Follow regulatory compliance guidelines, including HIPAA's Privacy and Security Rules.*

- *Generate statistical, aging, and financial analysis reports.*

Introduction

Electronic health records represent one of the biggest culture shifts in health care in the past several decades. While technology continues to expand into our lives, impacting how we shop, bank, and access entertainment, its impact on health care is significant. Not only has technology changed the way patients learn about health and disease, it has changed practice patterns, job responsibilities, and patient expectations in ways no one predicted, and will continue to exert an influence on the health care delivery system for the foreseeable future.

What is an electronic health record (EHR)? The concept of a computer-based patient record (CPR) was introduced in the 1980s when the Institute of Medicine (IOM) suggested that the implementation of computer technologies into managing health data would provide benefits unrealized to that point. Today the term electronic health record refers to the patient medical record that has transitioned away from paper and pen and into the cyber realm. For a more precise definition, the U.S. government has defined a qualified electronic health record as part of the language in the Health Information Technology for Economic and Clinical Health (HITECH) Act, which was introduced as part of the

American Recovery and Reinvestment Act (ARRA) of 2009. According to the HITECH Act, a qualified EHR must meet the following criteria:

- It must be an electronic record of health information that is specific to each individual.

- It must include patient demographic information.

- It must chronicle clinical information that would include a patient's medical history, as well as an on-going list of their health problems.

- It must provide clinical decision support (CDS).

- It must accommodate the addition of computerized provider (physician) order entry (CPOE).

- It must have the ability to store data and information specific to health care quality and provide functionality to retrieve this information through queries or other reporting functions.

- The EHR must allow for the exchange of electronic health information, including information from non-EHR (external) sources.

Under this umbrella of requirements, a number of EHR solutions have been developed, marketed, and sold and are in use across the health care delivery system today. In some cases, the terms EHR and EMR, or electronic medical record, are used interchangeably, and can cause confusion. To address the issue, the distinction is usually made between an EHR, which can be deployed across multiple health care facilities and meets national-recognized interoperability standards, and an electronic medical record (EMR), which is less concretely defined. The term EMR most often refers to an electronic system of health information that is confined to one facility. Generally, you will find EHRs deployed in hospitals and across a health system, and an EMR in use within a provider's office. The terms EHR and EMR will be used throughout this study guide to denote either hospitals or health systems (EHR) or providers' offices (EMR), which differ in their scope of practice and use of the technology.

Many articles and textbooks refer to "the EHR" as if it is a standard, single entity. The EHR is a concept that multiple companies and agencies continue to develop and refine to meet their own business goals. Therefore, an EHR in one hospital may not resemble in any form the EHR in the hospital across town, and in fact, the EHRs may not even be able to "talk to each other," or exchange information without some human intervention.

After reading this study guide, you will have the skills necessary to access information contained within an EHR or EMR and use this emerging technology as a tool to support the clinical staff in your facility in providing high quality patient care.

After taking an approved course of study, you are eligible to take a certification exam. You may be able to find employment without certification, but you will be competing against candidates who have obtained their certification. Certification is the standard in almost all medical and medical-related professions. Obtaining certification lets employers know you have demonstrated the knowledge necessary for competent practice.

This study guide prepares you for the Certified Electronic Health Records Specialist (CEHRS) exam the National Healthcareer Association (NHA) offers.

To be eligible to earn an NHA certification, you must possess either a high school diploma or its equivalency, and you must complete a training program or provide written proof that you have 1 year of work experience within the field. If you meet these criteria, you may register for the exam online at http://www.nhanow.com/health-record.aspx.

The CEHRS exam consists of 110 multiple-choice questions, with 100 of those items being scored. If your school is a registered NHA test site, you may take a proctored exam via computer or in paper-pencil format. You also have the option to take the exam via computer at a PSI testing center. You are allotted 110 minutes to complete the exam. You must achieve a scaled score of 390 out of 500 to pass the exam. Exam scores are sent to your home address about 3 to 5 business days after NHA receives your completed answer sheet.

Each chapter of this study guide begins with a list of learning objectives that introduces the concepts contained within the chapter. The key instructional content, or body of each chapter, follows the CEHRS test plan, which can be found before the first chapter. Following the key instructional content, you will find a chapter summary, which recaps the main points within the chapter; drill questions, which assess your knowledge of the chapter subjects; and a terms and definitions section, which defines the bolded words within the chapter.

Chapter 1: Software Applications and Equipment

The first chapter is broken into two sections: application operation and practice management. The application operation section explains how to manage backup of EHR data, retrieve patient information from the EHR database, and operate integrated devices with EHR software, such as scanners, fax machines, and cameras. The practice management section teaches you how to coordinate patient flow within the office, provide end-user training and technical support of EHR software, and edit existing searchable databases.

Chapter 2: Insurance and Billing

As an EHR specialist, you should understand the insurance and billing process. Chapter 2 first introduces how to enter codes and billing information into an EHR. It also explains abstracting diagnoses and procedures from the medical record, as well as generating patient statements, encounter forms, superbills, and admission sheets. Lastly, you will learn how to locate codes in the ICD-10-CM, ICD-10-PCS, CPT, and HCPCS coding manuals.

Chapter 3: Charting

Charting, or documenting patient care, is an important task in paper or electronic medical records. Clinical staff document the care they provide to patients so the data is available to support consistent, quality care for each patient. The data is also important for reporting on quality measures, supporting research and education, and developing improvements to care. Monitoring patient records in the electronic environment is an important aspect of your job as a certified EHR specialist, as well as working to ensure that the data within them are accurate, secure, and complete.

Chapter 3 describes the different data sources which populate an EHR and it outlines your role in file maintenance procedures, such as purging, archiving, and finalizing. This chapter also details how to audit charts to ensure compliance with the various regulatory and accreditation agencies and documents the link between accurate documentation and reimbursement.

Chapter 4: Regulatory Compliance

As a health care worker, it is important that you understand and abide by the requirements set forth by the Health Insurance Portability and Accountability Act (HIPAA) as well as the additional regulations outlined in the HITECH Act. Personal responsibility for protecting and safeguarding the protected health information (PHI) of patients whose information you have access to is no longer just a professional courtesy – it is required by federal law and individuals who fail to abide by the regulations can face steep fines and even jail time. Chapter 4 describes best practices in maintaining the confidentiality of PHI, as well as how to detect and reconcile threats to the security of electronic information. You will also learn about internal audits of medical records and how to execute a data recovery plan should a catastrophic event occur.

Chapter 5: Reporting

Another benefit of EHRs is the ability to generate robust reports. Chapter 5 introduces using the data available in an EHR or EMR to generate statistical reports for clinical and financial quality improvement (QI) measures, aging reports by guarantor or insurance carrier, and financial analysis reports by provider, diagnosis, or procedure. Reports by specific disease or patient type can be queried from an EHR and provide value to on-going performance improvement initiatives and more.

Case Studies

Following the chapters, there are three scenarios that test your accumulated knowledge in all areas of the study guide. Each scenario represents a real-life situation and requires critical thinking skills to effectively complete the discussion questions that follow.

NHA Certified Electronic Health Record Specialist (CEHRS) 2011 Detailed Test Plan 100 scored items, 10 pretest items	# scored items
1. Software Applications and Equipment	**24**
A. Application Operation	**12**
1. Manage backup of EHR data (e.g., restore patient data).	
2. Execute EHR work flows within a healthcare facility (e.g., clinical and administrative protocols).	
3. Retrieve patient information from the EHR database.	
4. Store patient information in the EHR database.	
5. Acquire external patient data.	
6. Edit EHR with proper privileges.	
7. Perform routine EHR clinical and/or administrative tasks within a healthcare facility per facility protocols.	
8. Transmit patient data for external use (e.g., insurance, pharmacies, other providers).	
9. Execute software updates.	
10. Maintain inventory of software and hardware assets.	
11. Operate integrated devices with EHR software (e.g., scanners, fax machine, signature pads, cameras).	
12. Access clinical vocabularies in a health information system when appropriate.	
B. Practice Management	**12**
1. Maintain a provider database for the purpose of continuity of care.	
2. Develop clinical templates for data capture (e.g., by diagnosis, by procedure, by practice).	
3. Coordinate patient flow within the office (e.g., scheduling, patient registration and verification, patient referrals).	
4. Provide ongoing end-user training of EHR software.	

NHA Certified Electronic Health Record Specialist (CEHRS) 2011 Detailed Test Plan 100 scored items, 10 pretest items	# scored items
5. Provide end-user technical support of EHR software.	
6. Edit existing searchable databases (e.g., code changes, patient demographics, insurance carriers).	
7. Identify inconsistencies between patient information and practice management software.	
2. Insurance and Billing	**20**
A. Enter coding and billing information in the EHR.	
B. Abstract diagnoses and procedural descriptions from the medical record.	
C. Enter diagnoses and procedural descriptions from the medical record into the EHR.	
D. Generate insurance verification reports.	
E. Generate patient statements.	
F. Post payments to patient accounts at the time of visit.	
G. Generate encounter forms/superbills.	
H. Generate face/admission sheets.	
I. Find codes in the ICD, CPT, and HCPCS manuals.	
3. Charting	**25**
A. Monitor the provider documentation for completeness and accuracy.	
B. Categorize patient's health information into a reliable and organized system that promotes error identification.	
C. Enter live data into an EHR.	
D. Assist clinicians with charting.	
E. Locate requested information in a patient chart.	

NHA Certified Electronic Health Record Specialist (CEHRS) 2011 Detailed Test Plan 100 scored items, 10 pretest items	# scored items
F. Execute file maintenance procedures (e.g., purging, archiving, finalizing, securing).	
G. Audit charts to ensure compliance of proper charting.	
H. Document the link between effective charting and reimbursement for procedures performed by clinicians.	
4. Regulatory Compliance	**21**
A. Adhere to professional standards of care as they pertain to medical records.	
B. Maintain confidentiality of Protected Health Information (PHI) in compliance with HIPAA Privacy Rule and facility policy.	
C. Maintain security of Protected Health Information (PHI) in compliance with HIPAA Security Rule and facility policy.	
D. Detect threats to the security of electronic information.	
E. Reconcile threats to the security of electronic information.	
F. Audit compliance and report to proper enforcement officer.	
G. Release Protected Health Information (PHI) in accordance with HIPAA and facility policy.	
H. Participate in internal audits of medical records (e.g., consent forms, Release of Information forms (ROI), signature on file).	
I. Comply with patient safety standards regarding abbreviations in a health information system.	
J. Execute a plan for data recovery in the case of a catastrophic event.	
K. De-identify Protected Health Information (PHI) when directed.	

NHA Certified Electronic Health Record Specialist (CEHRS) 2011 Detailed Test Plan 100 scored items, 10 pretest items	# scored items
5. Reporting	**10**
A. Generate statistical reports for clinical Quality Improvement (QI) measures.	
B. Compile medical care and census data for continuity of care records (e.g., statistical reports on diseases treated, surgery performed, use of hospital beds for clinical audits).	
C. Generate statistical reports for financial Quality Improvement (QI) measures.	
D. Generate aging reports by guarantor or carrier.	
E. Generate financial analysis reports by provider, diagnosis, or procedure.	

01 SOFTWARE APPLICATIONS AND EQUIPMENT

Learning Objectives

After reading this chapter, you will be able to:

- *Manage backup of EHR data.*

- *Execute EHR workflows within a facility.*

- *Retrieve patient information from the EHR database.*

- *Store patient information in the EHR database.*

- *Acquire external patient data.*

- *Edit the EHR with proper privileges.*

- *Perform routine EHR clinical and administrative tasks within a facility per facility protocols.*

- *Transmit patient data for external use, such as for insurance companies, pharmacies, and other providers.*

- *Execute software updates.*

- *Maintain inventory of software and hardware assets.*

- *Operate integrated devices with EHR software, such as scanners, fax machines, signature pads, and cameras.*

- *Access clinical vocabularies in a health information system when appropriate.*

- *Maintain a provider database for the purpose of continuity of care.*

- *Develop clinical templates for data capture, such as by diagnosis, by procedure, or by practice.*

- *Coordinate patient flow within the office, such as scheduling, patient registration and verification, and patient referrals.*

- *Provide ongoing end-user training and end-user support of EHR software.*

- *Edit existing searchable databases.*

- *Identify inconsistencies between patient information and practice management software.*

Introduction

EHR specialists work with important patient data using computers and information systems. They must abide by federal and state laws, as well as regulatory and accreditation agency requirements for the handling of patient information, and stay up to date on the emerging trends in technology and regulation. Providers, nurses, and other health care professionals rely on the skills of support staff to maintain patient data, which in turn supports continued, high-quality patient care.

Health care professionals can use the terms electronic records, **electronic health records (EHRs)**, and **electronic medical records (EMRs)** interchangeably because they generally mean the same thing. The federal government calls it **EHR technology**. This technology includes large, integrated EHR systems and smaller, single-use EMR software. To get you accustomed to the many uses of each term, this study guide uses EHR to refer to hospitals and EMR to refer to provider offices. It is important to understand there is no single "EHR." This term represents a concept that manifests through various hardware and software applications from various and competing facilities.

This study guide introduces you to the basics of managing data processes in the EHR environment in both inpatient and outpatient settings.

APPLICATION OPERATION

Manage Backup of EHR Data

The EMR and EHR contain important clinical and patient information. Your role includes keeping this data safe from destruction, ensuring it is available for clinician use, and making sure it stays private and secure. Early in the evolution of technology in the workplace – health care and otherwise – normal backup procedures involved an appointed person running a day-end process to copy all the day's transactions and data to a magnetic disk and storing this off-site, whether someone in the office takes it home or has a service pick it up. Today's increasingly complex information systems along with the emerging legal and ethical implications that accompany the storage of **protected health information (PHI)** have made these practices less than ideal. Thankfully, technological advancements have improved the options for storage and disaster recovery of important patient, clinical, and business information.

Hospitals and larger facilities generally employ robust **information technology (IT) departments** staffed with professional IT experts who manage the storage, retrieval, and backup of data that is generated as a part of normal business operations. In a hospital or larger facility, data backup processes fall outside your job description. However, all personnel who access and use an information system need to be well-versed in the policies and procedures for protecting data across the enterprise. As such, they should practice good data and information management habits, including observing the user ID and password guidelines at your facility by not sharing passwords, logging out when leaving your computer, and avoiding cyber behaviors that can put your system at risk, such as downloading external content or plugging an unknown USB drive into the system. Regular and open communication between the **Health Information Management (HIM) departments** and IT department can help avoid data disasters.

Small clinic or provider offices may still opt to manage data backup and recovery using magnetic tapes or similar download and storage options, but you must consider protecting the patient and business data.

Magnetic tapes do not last forever. To ensure quality results, test your backup tapes regularly to ensure data integrity and availability. Having a system that works perfectly on paper is no substitute for a system that is fool-proof as a result of regular testing. Schedule regular test restores from the tapes to make sure that, if needed, you can restore the system to its full functionality. Having a process that has never been tested is as risky as having no plan.

Be sure that if your facility uses tapes, it stores them at an off-site location. Ideally, this would be in a geographically distant location that can avoid local disasters, such as fires, floods, tornados, or other threatening events.

Some smaller facilities may opt for a web-based EMR system that allows access to the software and system functionality through thin-client technology. This allows local access to the software and data in the EMR, but all records and information remain on a remote server off-site. The system vendor accepts responsibility for data backup, protection, and recovery in case of a disaster. **Health Insurance Portability and Accountability (HIPAA) Privacy** and **Security rules** fall under the guidelines for business associates. Business associates are required to adhere to HIPAA regulations as outlined in the original HIPAA legislation and further delineated in the **Health Information Technology for Economic and Clinical Health (HITECH) Act**.

Some provider offices may opt to use an EMR that is not web-based and store their data in a remote hosting facility. These sites provide a secure portal where you upload the data at the end of the day. Just like the web-based EMR products, these companies are considered business associates are held to the same HIPAA and HITECH Act standards for safeguarding PHI.

The **American Recovery and Reinvestment Act of 2009 (ARRA)** introduced increased responsibilities and greater punishments for improper management of PHI. **Covered entities**, including hospitals, provider offices, and clinics, as well as their **business associates**, which are often known as third-party vendors, are responsible for proper handling of PHI and are accountable for any breach of information or privacy. Providers should exercise care in selecting data backup or storage solutions to abide by the legal requirements established under HIPAA and the HITECH Act in the protection of the patient's most personal and private information.

Execute EHR Workflows within a Health Care Facility

Inpatient workflow as it relates to the EHR is more complex and involves multiple scenarios as compared to the outpatient workflow. In the inpatient environment, it is common to find many **legacy information systems** that predate EHR implementation and represent a variety of companies or vendors. It is not unusual to find hospitals with pharmacy, radiology, laboratory, and registration systems that originated from unrelated vendors. Although many companies now manufacture total health IT solutions, many combinations of information systems remain in use within hospitals today. Imagine the cost and the disruption to daily operations when a hospital decides to tear out all existing information systems and install a single solution. While this does happen in some facilities, it is extremely expensive and disruptive. Think about the last time you had to update the version of software you use. Now, imagine how much bigger that adjustment would be when applied across a hospital or health system.

When the total solution is not the answer, hospitals will add component systems to their existing IT infrastructure. This requires the work of IT professionals and experts in interoperability and data exchange standards. In the U.S. health care delivery system, the data exchange standards most often referenced include the following:

- American National Standard Institute (ANSI) Accredited Standards Committee X12 (ASC X12)

- The American Society for Testing and Materials (ASTM)

- Digital Imaging and Communications in Medicine (DICOM)

- Health Level Seven (HL7)

- National Council for Prescription Drug Programs (NCPDP)

Different health information systems that wish to communicate with each other must adhere to the standards set forth by these organizations.

Patients present to an inpatient admission in several ways. They may arrive at the emergency department (ED) as an emergency case. They may schedule a surgery based on recommendations from a provider. Or, their provider may admit them after an office visit. The EHR workflow varies somewhat from facility to facility, but always begins with registration and entering the patient's demographic data into the EHR system and identifying them as an active patient. As an EHR specialist, you may work in the patient registration department of a hospital. Your primary job would focus on the proper identification and documentation of the patient's personal and financial information, mainly his insurance. This information allows the facility to bill for the services they provide.

In the inpatient environment, the provider inputs an admission order into the EHR system, using the **Computerized Provider Order Entry (CPOE)** module. After the provider enters the admission order, he can also order the patient's diet, any medications, tests, including laboratory or imaging studies, and what are commonly referred to as **patient care orders (PCOs)** or nursing orders. PCOs specify if the patient can be out of bed without assistance, how often nurses complete dressing changes, and other care that the provider orders and nurses perform. During the hospital admission stay, the various clinicians providing care document a patient's course of care. The majority of the charting, meaning the inpatient documentation in the EHR, is nursing and physician notes. **The Joint Commission on the Accreditation of Health Care Organizations (Joint Commission)** and the **Centers for Medicare and Medicaid Services (CMS)** require that the patient record contain a current **History and Physical (H and P)** report within 24 hr of the patient's admission. A patient who undergoes any surgical procedures will also have an anesthesia report, operative report, and pathology report if a surgeon removes any tissue during the procedure. If a physician consults other physicians about a patient's care, the provider uses CPOE to enter a consultation order into the EHR. Once the consulting physician sees the patient and can add his expertise to the patient's condition, he writes a report on the findings, which then appears in the patient's record as a consult.

Throughout the inpatient stay, results from imaging studies, such as ultrasound, computed tomography (CT), magnetic resonance imaging (MRI), basic radiological (x-ray) studies, and positron emission tomography (PET) scans, are available in the EHR due to interoperability functions that allow the radiology and laboratory systems to share their data with the EHR system. In many facilities, the laboratory, radiology, and pharmacy information systems have been in place since the 1980s. EHRs are relatively new in terms of active use in the hospital environment, so a great deal of work preceded linking these older systems with the new EHR and CPOE systems.

The ability of different systems to communicate is made possible when all systems use the accepted industry standards, such as HL7, and interface software that provides the linkage between, for example, a pharmacy system and an EHR. This is necessary so the medication details the provider ordered using CPOE can be received in the pharmacy information system, and then processed, reviewed, and documented. Once the order is processed, appropriately verified, and prepared for patient administration, the pharmacy information system can then send the information back across the interface to populate the patient record in the EHR system. As the nurse administers the medication, all details are accurately documented in the patient record.

Patients often participate in physical, speech, or occupational therapy sessions. These professionals also document patient progress in the EHR in the area specific to rehabilitation. Test results from blood work or other laboratory diagnostics transmit automatically from the laboratory information system into the patient record within the EHR so physicians, nurses, and other personnel, such as therapists or pharmacists, can access the data and use the data to make treatment or care decisions – whereas technicians and technologists who perform the tests enter the tests in the laboratory information system. Much of the laboratory testing is batch processed and feeds from the automated analytical instrument that performs the testing into the laboratory information system, which then interfaces with the EHR system to distribute the results. When all systems are functioning as expected, this process happens seamlessly and without human intervention.

In the inpatient environment, your role varies depending on the maturity of the EHR system in place. For hospitals on the early side of adopting EHR technology, opportunities to train clinical staff in the use of the EHR system will be plentiful, whereas in more mature facilities that have been using EHR technology for some time, the role of training becomes less prominent and is often tasked to the internal education department. You may find opportunities in the HIM department where reporting functions originate based on the data and information stored in the EHR. Recent legislation on **meaningful use** and the expanding requirements by accrediting agencies for the documentation of quality patient care require careful analysis and reporting.

The outpatient provider office or small clinic workflows are much less complex than the inpatient workflows. In many provider office settings, a single software program manages the appointment, registration, and patient care documentation activities. If you work in an outpatient setting, you may find a role that includes scheduling patients, checking them in before their appointments, and assisting the clinical staff in the documentation of the patient care they provide. In some situations, you may also be asked to assist with coding or billing activities, depending on your knowledge, experience, and the needs of the office.

Retrieve Patient Information from the EHR Database

EHR specialists possess excellent skills for the extraction of data and information from an EHR or EMR system. Physicians and other clinical staff members, such as medical assistants, document the various patient care items in the EMR as they provide care. When appropriate, you can provide coaching or what is known as at-the-elbow technical support for the clinical staff using the EMR for the first time. This immediate availability of support encourages quicker adoption and use of EHR technology when introducing it into a clinical environment.

You can provide important assistance by pointing out how the various tools in the EMR, including templates, clinical alerts, and available knowledge databases, such as the **Physician's Desk Reference (PDR)**, are available at the click of a mouse. When a physician uses the EMR to its full capacity, she has the opportunity to provide important reports that support patients' health, assist the facility in meeting regulatory and legal requirements, and generally enhance the work that occurs in the office or clinic.

Preventative care data presents one example of reporting you can accomplish based on data a provider enters into the EMR. Insurers and physicians alike remain interested in preventing disease before it creates patient dysfunction. In an effort to support this, federal legislation in the form of the **Affordable Care Act** requires that Medicare patients receive an annual physical examination. Most physical exams include basic health screenings to detect disease states as early as possible. These screenings include a fecal occult blood test to detect colorectal cancer; cholesterol; blood testing for early detection of hyperlipidemia or diabetes; colonoscopies; mammograms; and prostate exams. A physician's office is interested in maintaining optimal health for its patients. Therefore, you will need to create reports based on the data in the EMR for active patients. You can create a regular assessment report on the health status of a patient by querying the EMR database. This report could be annual, quarterly, or monthly. Data from laboratory and radiology tests populate the patient record in the EMR through staff input or by automatic transmission. As federal incentives and legislation continue to drive the EHR and EMR world toward discrete or structured data (as opposed to free text data), reporting becomes easier. You can set up a query to find all of the 40-year-old female patients to see if there is documentation of a mammogram in their record. You can also generate a report to identify patients age 50 and older who do not have documentation of a colonoscopy screening procedure. In highly-integrated environments, the computer can print out reminder letters or send automatic emails to patients without a test on record. In less digitized environments, the office staff may need to manually send reminders to those without a test on record.

You can also provide important real-time data to a provider or clinical staff for patient visits. Managing diabetic patients remains a challenge for some providers. With regular documentation of blood glucose levels in the patient record, stored as discrete data in the EMR, you can prepare special or ad hoc reports for the clinician to show a patient's blood glucose levels over time, information much more valuable in making a clinical decision than a single blood glucose value at the time of the office visit. Recalls on prescription medications, medical devices, and implanted devices remain relatively common. EMR data proves invaluable in identifying those patients at risk from a recalled pharmaceutical or other item. A simple query written to return all patients who were prescribed the medication or provided with the medical device can save hours of time as compared to searching through paper-based records.

Store Patient Information in the EHR Database

Since the inception of medical recordkeeping in the early part of the 20th century, standardization of documentation in acute care or inpatient records – regardless of whether the records are paper-based or electronic – requires each record to include the following:

- Patient demographic or registration information

- Patient medical history

- Physical examination of the patient

    - The medical history combined with the physical exam is known as H and P.

- Clinical data and observations

    - Progress notes that physicians, nurses, and any therapists providing care or treatment document are included in this section.

- Physician orders

- Result reports from diagnostic testing and therapeutic procedures

    - These reports include laboratory results and imaging study conclusions.

- Consultations

    - Consultations are reports from a physician to whom the patient has been referred for a second or specialty opinion.

- Discharge summary

- Patient instructions

- Acknowledgements, **authorizations**, and consent forms

Be sure the data contained within the EHR is up to date and meets accreditation and regulatory standards. Remember, the Joint Commission requires that each patient record contain a current H and P within 24 hr of admission. CMS requires that the physician file and sign the **discharge summary** within 30 days of discharge. Paper and electronic records with missing provider signatures are considered incomplete. Facilities with too many incomplete records receive negative findings in a Joint Commission survey site visit or a CMS audit. CMS requires facilities that treat and bill for Medicare and Medicaid patients meet certain **Conditions of Participation (CoPs)** which are similar to the requirements set forth by the Joint Commission. In recent years, the Joint Commission and CMS have partnered, so hospitals and other facilities can avoid double work. CMS considers any facility that has Joint Commission accreditation status to be a "deemed" facility, meaning the facility also meets CMS requirements and does not need a separate distinct process and site visit to verify that they meet the CoPs.

Making sure all required data is present, appropriate, accurate, and authenticated is an important records management task. This means the proper clinical staff signed and dated the data as required by law. Missing data not only puts patients at risk, but places the facility in jeopardy of losing accreditation or losing its deemed status from CMS. Loss of status results in the inability to treat Medicare and Medicaid patients, which in some facilities represents more than 50% of the business.

Record components remain basically the same in the outpatient or ambulatory setting. Clinical staff document patient demographics, medical history, and physical examinations in much the same way as they do in the inpatient setting. Differences in the outpatient record reflect the care pattern differences, such as tracking growth of pediatric patients, documenting vaccines, immunizations, and preventive care activities, such as annual mammograms and prostate screenings. The outpatient record also includes a problem list, which is an ever-present listing of the patient's issues, so at each visit, the clinician can acknowledge and consider the concurrent issues in the treatment of the presenting problem. For example, a patient who has type 2 diabetes mellitus and was involved in a motor vehicle accident and has a abrasion on his lower right leg that the provider is watching and treating weekly. Patients who have diabetes mellitus frequently have challenges around wound healing. The problem list reminds the clinician the patient has diabetes to ensure the best assessment and treatment options are made for the patient. In busy provider offices or clinics where patients may see a different provider each week, the problem list helps patient care remain focused on the whole patient, resulting in higher quality outcomes.

Problem lists are also a requirement in the acute care record for hospitals, but the implementation and use remains a challenge. Questions remain on how many problems should populate the list and how many historical problems should be listed. Acute care is episodic, so while a patient's diabetes is relevant to almost every medical encounter, a history of migraine headaches may not be important to the current episode of care. Sorting through what makes sense to include in the acute record problem list and when to include the information remains a discussion for hospital administrators, legislators, and, ultimately, accreditation and regulatory agencies.

Acquire External Patient Data

Patients create data each time they interface with the health care delivery system. This data often resides outside of the hospital or provider's office where the patient's record exists. Directing all of the information into each patient's electronic record presents challenges to completely and thoroughly document the patient's experience.

The simplest option for integrating external data into the patient's EMR is scanning the documents and uploading the images into the record. Scanning is better than having no record of external health care episodes. However, the disadvantage to this method is that the data does not reside as discrete, or structured, data – it's only as part of a scanned image or document.

Technological advancements in the sharing of health data have improved the ability of external information to integrate with electronic records. The **Continuity of Care Record** (**CCR**) served as the solution initially, but this concept has evolved into the

Continuity of Care Document (**CCD**). The CCD is now the standard for a number of reasons, one of which being it is a federal government mandate for facilities that are participating in the financial incentives to adopt EHR technology by achieving meaningful use.

The CCD represents the industry standard for the transmission of health data between providers, such as hospital to clinician or clinician to clinician. In 2008, the **Certification Commission for Health Information Technology** (**CCHIT**) endorsed the CCD as the preferred continuity of care format for certified EHR products. By design, the CCD contains specific elements from the patient record that providers agree are the most relevant to continuity of patient care, including current and previous health information. The CCD is also specifically designed for accessibility by any computer system, application, or EHR or EMR system. This provides its intended benefit: patient information sharing across care environments. EHR specialists play an important role in supporting quality health care when they manage the sending and receiving of CCDs in hospitals, clinics, and providers' offices.

Patients often have a history of multiple providers in various geographic locations and individual records for each provider, most of them still in paper-based format. This presents a challenge for their current provider because past medical history is important to the management of patients' health, especially with chronic disease. While new options exist for the sharing of data generated in EHR systems, the options for incorporating paper-based medical history into an electronic records system remain fairly simple. Document imaging of paper records remains the industry practice, but it has limitations. How much of patients' old records do providers need or want in the current electronic record? How should they determine what to **digitize** and what to store in a traditional **off-site location**? Record management companies offer multiple solutions to these challenges, and each facility and department decides what works best for their facility and patients. You can participate on a committee that investigates the best options for the department or facility and, in partnership with the clinical staff, can provide valuable insights into which solution meets the most needs for providers and patients alike.

Edit EHR with Proper Privileges

When performing edits in the EHR environment, you must take into consideration the regulations governing record documentation, as well as software capabilities and the appropriateness of the edits.

You should never alter or edit patient care documentation a provider enters into a patient's record. If you have a concern about a specific data entry or documentation in a patient record, ask the person whose signature appears on the information about the issue.

It is unlawful to delete information from the patient record, as it is a legal record of the business activities for the facility. Erroneous or incorrect entries must remain in the record, with the new or correct data appearing as an addendum or correction note. Different software packages offer different options for making amendments, corrections, or additions, also known as late entries, to the record. The facility's policy and procedure for making corrections, addendums, and late entries is developed by an HIM professional in consultation with the clinical staff and in consideration of the software capabilities and limitations. You may be asked to participate in the development of, or update to, the existing policy. You can provide important quality assurance to the integrity of the patient record by maintaining your knowledge on the policy and helping the clinical staff to remember to practice proper documentation techniques.

Perform Routine EHR Clinical and/or Administrative Tasks per Facility Protocols

Your responsibilities will vary based on the environment you work in, the patient population your facility serves, the component makeup of other staff members, and the preference of the management team for who performs which tasks.

In a hospital or inpatient environment, you will likely be employed within the HIM department or IT department, depending on what other skills you possess and how the hospital is organized for the management of the EHR. Your role in either of these departments hinges largely on the tasks each department performs. In some hospitals and health systems, these departments work together but are separate in terms of their work. For example, the IT department handles all the technology issues, whereas HIM personnel stay strictly involved with the administration of patient records. In other facilities, this boundary is less clear and the HIM and IT departments work closely to manage the EHRs and other aspects of the hospital information system.

In a traditional HIM department where there is minimal IT crossover work, your role as an EHR specialist may include duties such as retrieving records, microfilm, or information from electronic records as requested by accessing the appropriate information system. You will likely need to prepare records and any paper sheet documentation by filing, scanning, microfilming, or indexing. Because most hospitals and health care systems are not functioning as fully-integrated electronic environments, the likelihood is quite high that you will work with a hybrid record. A hybrid record environment is one where there is an electronic records system of some level, but paper records are also maintained. The mix of what is paper and what is electronic is not the same in any facility, and figuring out what constitutes the legal health record remains a challenge in these facilities. Therefore, many of your work tasks will span traditional medical records work as well as emerging EHR practices.

Performing quality checks on records and assembling requests for a copy of the legal health record in response to accreditation reviews or subpoenas may also fall under your responsibilities. You must learn to work with your facility's **Master Patient**

Index (**MPI**), an index that requires great attention to detail to preserve accuracy and completeness of patient information. In the hybrid environment, you may also track all patient records that leave the HIM department, as well as those that return by use of an electronic chart tracking system.

In an IT role, your work might focus more on using EHR applications, training others in their EHR use, and testing. It helps to have an IT background to enter this type of job because many of these jobs involve complex information systems tasks.

In an outpatient or provider office setting, these tasks are similar. You will need to incorporate record tracking, scanning, microfilming, and MPI maintenance into the rest of the office workflow, which will vary depending on the practice preferences and available staff.

Transmit Patient Data for External Use

Hospitals and physician offices also send data to other providers and facilities. You may find this is a regular part of your work day. In a hospital or health system, this role most often falls to the HIM department where there is a designated **release of information** (**ROI**) area. In an outpatient or clinic setting, this is likely a task for you.

Working in the ROI area requires that you be up to date in all the legal and regulatory guidelines for releasing PHI. HIPAA mandates that covered entities limit the amount of PHI they release.

In certain circumstances, you can release PHI without special authorization. These reasons include to support treatment, to seek reimbursement for services rendered, or to support the daily business operations of the facility. Federal, state, and local laws require that covered entities release PHI in response to subpoenas, legitimate law enforcement inquiries, and in cases of suspected abuse or neglect. Public health law also requires the reporting of sexually transmitted diseases. You may also release PHI in support of regulatory reviews, such as visits by the Joint Commission or CMS.

A patient must specifically authorize most other release of patient information. This authorization can also come from a legal representative, such as a family member with power of attorney, or in the case of a child, her parent or guardian. The authorization must be in writing and specific to what information she is allowing your facility to release. For example, the patient could write "Details of my hospitalization from May 30, 2009 through June 11, 2009." The authorization must detail who may release the information – naming the specific facility or provider – and who may receive it. It must also have a date when the authorization expires. It is important to note that an authorization to release a patient's PHI is not transferrable. For example, if a patient signs a release of information authorization at the hospital to have her surgery records sent to a provider's office, no one may re-release these same records to another provider practice or hospital even if her authorization has not expired. Privacy and security of patients' PHI is extremely important. When in doubt, ask before releasing any information.

Execute Software Updates

In hospitals and larger clinics and health systems, software updates are tasked to the internal IT department. How the internal IT department manages the implementation across the enterprise is unique to the preferences and structure of each facility.

In some facilities, IT security is very tight and no one except mid-level to senior IT analysts possess the appropriate administrative rights to make changes to applications. In other facilities, the IT department will grant administrative rights to users for specific tasks that may include updating software. In an era of increasing scrutiny and concern around protecting valuable patient information, restricting access to software updates or changes to applications is common. If you work in an IT department, this may fall under your scope of duties. Otherwise, the IT department may appoint a primary contact to serve as the liaison between the two departments. This responsibility may involve ensuring that each user logs off of his workstation when he leaves, but keeps the machine remaining on and not shut down completely to allow for after-hours updates. Enterprise-wide software solutions are also changing the workflow from requiring an installation on every PC or workstation to a process that the IT department can implement from the server and distribute across the network simultaneously.

In a smaller environment, such as a provider's office or small clinic, your role in updating software may range from extensive to minimal. With the CMS requirement that facilities applying to participate in the meaningful use incentive program have a certified EHR product, providers are avoiding the homegrown EHR solutions that at one time presented low-tech and affordable solutions.

Since 2006, CCHIT has been certifying EHR products. Using a certified EHR product was once an option – today it is essential. The meaningful use incentive program CMS launched in 2011 offers financial incentives for providers and hospitals to show they are using certified EHR technology in a meaningful way. The purpose of the reward program is to encourage the adoption of Health IT solutions so patient care is improved by the documented benefits of electronic systems. These benefits include a reduction in errors because of illegible handwriting or unavailable data, clinical alerts that can stop a medication error before the pharmacy dispenses a prescription, patient reminders that assist providers in keeping patients on medically-appropriate schedules for refill medications, testing, or other interventions, and clinical decision support, which provides real time cause and effect feedback when a medical decision is under consideration. The incentives are significant. Eligible professionals, such as providers in a private practice can receive up to $44,000 over 5 years for seeing Medicare patients or up to $63,750, for seeing Medicaid patients, and demonstrating meaningful use of a certified EHR system. For hospitals, the incentives total millions of dollars.

Smaller offices rely on vendor-driven EHR solutions. While there are smaller vendors that rely on in-house personnel for IT tasks and updates, it is likely that most EHR system updates are at least coordinated by the vendor or a professional IT service. As an EHR specialist, you may also be designated as the go-to person between the vendor and the users in the facility setting.

Depending on the level of IT support in your office or clinic, you may find non-EHR updates are included in your responsibilities. Be sure you are aware of software license laws and keep current with security issues, patches released by the software manufacturer, and compatibility issues among various applications. When in doubt, call an IT professional to assist. A lot is at stake in a facility that has patient information accessible online, and since the HITECH Act, individuals as well as facilities may be held liable for PHI breaches.

Maintain Inventory of Software and Hardware Assets

In hospitals and larger clinics, the IT department manages the inventory of software and hardware assets. You may be asked to assist by keeping data on the machines, peripherals, and other devices you use in your department. Most facilities employ an inventory tracking system that tags and identifies all capital equipment that is purchased. Using a spreadsheet application to log, track, and assign individuals to specific equipment, such as desktop computers, laptops, or pagers, is one way to stay organized and make any reporting requirements simple to manage. Be sure to check with your facility's IT department on their guidelines for inventory management.

In smaller clinics or provider offices, the maintenance of software and hardware assets may fall to an outside consulting firm, the office manager, or to you. In this role, you should keep a file, listing, or ledger of the equipment, software, and accessories that have been purchased for the facility's use. A simple database or spreadsheet can accommodate the needs of most small to mid-size facilities. For software, document the following:

- Software title
- Version
- Publisher
- Date acquired or purchased
- Total installations or number of PCs where it is installed

Also, document the number of licenses purchased for the software and collect information as to the type of license, such as upgrade, retail, open license, select license, enterprise agreement, or other. For hardware, when detailing computers include documentation of the employee, such as the employee's name or the employee's ID, along with the hardware description, such as tablet PC or desktop, and details on the CPU, RAM, and operating system. With the rise in laptops and handheld computers, including smart phones and tablets, this hardware list needs to expand to include any devices purchased for employee use.

Operate Integrated Devices with EHR Software

Computer technology allows users to integrate peripheral devices, including printers, scanners, and cameras. In health care, the move away from paper-based transactions to electronic systems has ushered in new devices to capture signatures, provide documentation of patient identity, ensure medication safety, and replace paper processes that have ceased to be efficient or safe.

In a hospital or larger clinic environment, the level of device penetration closely follows the level of EHR integration throughout the system. In a **fully-integrated EHR** environment, you'll find more instances of electronic capture of information and that paper records only exist as previous records. Electronic signature pads capture patients' acknowledgements, receipt of privacy policies, consents for treatment, and responsibility for any charges. In some facilities, the patient may sign in to the waiting room using a computer. This enables you to preload some basic demographic data before the patient is called to the front desk. Small card scanners can scan the front then the back of insurance cards and return verification or denial of coverage within minutes.

Hospitals in transition or in a hybrid record state may use fax technology to order prescriptions from the pharmacy until they have fully implemented a CPOE system. Providers can order the medications through the **hospital information system (HIS)** and print the order out on special paper to sign and fax to the pharmacy for processing. After the pharmacy processes the order, the HIM department receives, then scans the document into the patient record or electronic document management system for permanent placement.

Providers' offices use fax technology to send and receive patient information. They may use both traditional and eFax technology. Using a standard fax involves feeding a document through the fax machine and dialing a number so the image is sent to the intended destination. With eFax capability, the document is sent from the computer without activating the fax machine and it prints out on a traditional fax machine at its destination.

Camera technology is useful in health care for documenting physical ailments like rashes, lumps, or bumps and in cases of suspected abuse or assault where there is a legal need to document the patient's condition at the point of care. Surgical information systems include specialty cameras that can take microscopic and full-size photos to assist in documenting important findings and patient status. The inpatient use of photos in the electronic record varies in scope and use depending on the department. Patient photographs fall under the same privacy protections as written information. Handle photographs accordingly.

In the outpatient environment, documenting patients' physical presentations may require that you work with providers and other clinical staff to understand how to capture, save, and transmit the images into the EMR. Most EMR software allows image uploads. The process should not present major obstacles to staff members because it resembles attaching a file to email or uploading a photo to a social networking site. Some providers' offices or clinics may want to take their patients' photograph so they can remember who they are and provide more personalized customer service. If a patient is ever uncomfortable with this process, respect the request and do not force the issue.

Barcode scanners are one of the most useful peripheral devices in electronic records systems today. Bar code technology sets the standard for patient identification and the prevention of medical mistakes. Studies show that patient safety in hospitals improves when using armbands equipped with barcode technology to distinguish a patient's name or medical record number. Barcoded armbands assist in the identification of patients before medication administration and at the beginning of surgical or other invasive procedures, such as drawing blood for testing. Many hospitals use **Computers on Wheels** (**COW**s) or **Wireless on Wheels** (**WOW**s), which often include a handheld barcode scanner. When a nurse enters a patient room to give medication, he must ask the patient for her full name and date of birth or identify the patient in another way if the patient is unable to speak or the patient is an infant, and then scan the patient armband and verify in the computer that the information captured by the scanner matches the information provided by the patient or family. In addition, many pharmacy information system applications have integrated the barcode technology so prescription medications that are dispensed have a barcode on the back of the blister pack. To properly administer the medication and document it, the nurse must scan the armband of the patient and the barcode on the medication. Any deviation from the correct patient, dose, or time of administration results in an audible alert that requires intervention. In addition to error prevention, barcode technology makes charting easier. Once the nurse scans the medication and verifies it in the computer, his system log in status serves as the signature for the medication administration record. This prevents the nurse from walking out of the room, forgetting to document that a patient received her morphine dose at 9 p.m.

A similar use of barcode technology is available in the outpatient environment. Clinical staff can easily and accurately document vaccines and injections for pain, inflammation, or other treatment using the barcode scan process for EMR documentation.

Access Clinical Vocabularies in a Health Information System when Appropriate

Medical terminology is the language of medicine. However, it fails to account for the numerous vocabularies, classifications, nomenclatures, and other terminologies health care professionals rely on to effectively communicate important data and information.

The American Medical Association (AMA) publishes and maintains **Current Procedural Terminology (CPT)** codes, a nomenclature or naming system. These codes help document provider and outpatient activities for reimbursement purposes. **International Classification of Diseases, 10th Revision, Clinical Modification (ICD-10-CM)** ICD-10-CM is a classification system that groups diseases and disorders into similar categories. Use the ICD-10-CM manual to assign codes for reimbursement purposes. ICD-10-PCS codes describe procedures performed for hospital inpatients. The ICD-10-CM/PCS manuals provide a source of data used for continuous performance improvement studies, research, and education in health care.

The **Systematized Nomenclature of Medicine - Clinical Terms (SNOMED-CT)** is less prominent than CPT and ICD systems, though it is no less important. SNOMED-CT is the latest and most complete clinical vocabulary of the SNOMED versions. It provides a single, credible reference for medical terms. For providers in many facilities across diverse communities and locations, using a standardized vocabulary for medical terms is important. For example, it is important to know whether the "flu" listed in a patient record is caused by the influenza virus, and if so, is it influenza-A or influenza-B? If it is the influenza-A virus, is it of the H1N1 strain or the H3N2 strain? An ill patient cares little about the name of the virus, but to researchers, epidemiologists (those who track the cause of disease and how far it spreads and why), and providers, these are important details.

EHR technology enables linkages between these various vocabularies and nomenclatures in ways paper records could not. SNOMED-CT is mapped to ICD-10-CM/PCS, which means that when the provider selects an ICD-10-CM/PCS code after a patient encounter, there is a map that links that information to the SNOMED-CT term or terms. For an EHR or EMR system to become certified through CCHIT, it must be able to use ICD-10-CM/PCS or SNOMED-CT. Most systems provide clinical staff and other health care professionals with point-and-click access to these vocabularies and nomenclatures. EHR specialists who perform medical coding duties may need to access the actual vocabularies or terminologies, but every EHR specialist should learn how to access these references in their facility's system, and based on the needs of the clinical staff you work with, be able to explain how they work, why they are included in the system, and where to go to find more information.

Updates to reference libraries accessible in an EHR environment depend on the product. Many systems link to a website where the publisher manages the data remotely and a subscription maintains the provider's access to the data. Some facilities may opt to house the information internally and take on the responsibility of updating and maintaining the database themselves based on releases by the originating organization. In large academic medical centers and integrated delivery systems where a medical library is part of the core facility, the in-house option may be more viable. Smaller facilities and providers' offices may find the most cost-effective and efficient process to be the online subscription. Work with the clinical team to help them make the best decision that supports the facility's workflow and patient care processes.

PRACTICE MANAGEMENT

Maintain a Provider Database for the Purpose of Continuity of Care

Facilities are legally responsible for the providers they hire to care for patients. Physicians or medical staff receive appointments and privileges in the acute care environment. Although different models now exist since managed care emerged in the 1980s, many providers still practice medicine by maintaining privileges at various hospitals.

Privileges outline the activities a provider is permitted to engage in at a facility. For example, if a provider is granted privileges as an internal medicine physician, she could not deliver babies in the obstetrical unit. Granting privileges follows a process known as **credentialing**, which the HIM department often manages. You may help collect data on the physician, including education, medical license, specialty training and licensure, and appropriate background checks that include obtaining information from the **National Practitioner Data Bank** (**NPDB**). The Health Care Quality Improvement Act of 1986 established the NPDB to address bad physicians who were previously able to travel to a different state and work as a provider after losing their license in the previous state, with no follow-up documentation.

You may work on the data collection for credentialing, as well as manage the internal data for all credentialed past and present providers. You may also serve on the **Medical Staff committee** and provide valuable input and information to the committee, and ultimately the hospital board of directors.

In outpatient settings, standalone clinics are more likely to hire providers as employees than grant privileges. Your expertise may come into play in this process, although in this case, the hiring becomes more a human resources function than an organizational policy decision. Some physician offices exist as multi-provider facilities where there is a partner or associate relationship between the providers. Many others are smaller partnership or solo practice structures where credentialing would not be the process in place for adding new providers to the facility. Physician hiring practices at hospital-owned or affiliated outpatient clinics vary depending on the governance structure. As in any new job, learn the policies and procedures specific to your facility so you can provide the best services to your employer and patients.

Develop Clinical Templates for Data Capture

Clinical **templates** are predesigned forms that capture data in a pattern that is specific to the facility's workflow and to the specific tasks within the various workflows.

EHR systems found in the inpatient environment generally do not provide the opportunity for end users to create ad hoc templates. However, during the installation phase, consultants and technical experts from the EHR vendor are on-site to work with every department who will use the system to document workflow and develop templates that mirror the work as it unfolds throughout the day. You can provide important input to this process by serving on a team that documents clinical workflow and participates with the EHR implementation team in identifying and testing the new functionality.

In the outpatient setting, the availability of preloaded templates may be similar to the inpatient example above or your facility may purchase software that allows for some template modification post-install. Learning the options available to the end user is important. Before attempting to create templates in an existing system, check for appropriate permissions from a systems perspective. Keep all documentation and vendor contact information for future reference.

Clinical templates make the documentation experience easier while prompting physicians to include important data items. In the inpatient setting, admission assessments that prompt nurses to ask patients about allergies helps support proper patient care and ensures the facility is meeting the definition of meaningful use as it relates to the capture of patient allergies in the EHR. In the outpatient setting, you can add reminding patients about flu shots to the general office visit template. So even on a busy day, providers can remind each patient about this important preventive action.

EMR vendors are increasingly developing specialty EMR systems to meet the specific needs of facilities. This means a dermatologist's EMR software can have different templates than a family practice or pediatric practice and each can be tailored to meet the unique needs of the patient population of the facility. Your role is to learn your clinical staff and patients' needs and ensure the needs are met with a function in the EMR. If the needs are not met, be willing to do the research to learn what it takes to add the functionality and identify how it would benefit the facility and patients.

Clinical templates are also useful in creating letters for patients who need to miss work, go on light duty, submit a school absence excuse, and present proof of a physical exam. You can also create letters requesting a second opinion in template form, as well as letters to patients to report test results and remind them about late payments. Work with the EMR vendor to learn your facility's system and use it to improve the workflow for clinical staff, office staff, and patients.

Coordinate Patient Flow within the Office

In smaller outpatient settings, you will likely serve more than one role. While computer technology continues to streamline many tasks in business environments, there is still a need to coordinate and organize activities. Practice management software is common in smaller to medium-sized practice environments and it coordinates patient appointments, registration, insurance verification, and billing. Outside of health care, banking and businesses have longer histories of using technological solutions for business problems. Therefore, practice management software predates the implementation and widespread use of EMR systems.

Some facilities have standalone practice management software that functions outside of the EMR environment, while others will adopt a system that integrates products for all tasks. The functionality remains the same, although the access and use may vary by system and facility.

Regardless of the system setup, the task of managing the clerical workflow differs from the clinical workflow tasks in that the process and workflow remain fairly consistent with the paper-based processes. Instead of keeping a log or appointment book, log patient appointments using practice management software tools. Patients still provide insurance documentation that you can verify with the assistance of technological tools, such as web-based portals for insurance verification and card scanners to capture and store insurance card information for each patient.

Upon arrival at your facility, the patient presents to the reception area the same way, whether registration information is collected on paper or through a computer. Some offices now require patients to log in and populate preregistration information. Many older patients may find this more frustrating than helpful, but as the population that grew up with technology ages, this option will find its way into the culture of the office visit.

Patients continue to progress through basic business processes within hospitals and outpatient settings in a manner that seems little different from the past. If you work in an environment with other clerical staff of varying technical skill, you may have an opportunity to teach less technical colleagues how to incorporate, or even embrace, information technology into the clerical workflow of the facility.

The process for patient referrals and consultation requests does not change aside from the use of premade templates, which expedites the process and eliminate delays for the patient.

Provide Ongoing End-user Training of EHR Software

One of the most important tasks in an increasingly technical health care environment is the end-user support function. Your expert knowledge about the functions and processes to enter and navigate complex systems provide valuable at-the-elbow coaching for clinical staff members who are often frustrated in making the transition from paper-based to electronic records. Research on provider adoption of EHR technology has shown they learn best with one-on-one coaching, not in a classroom environment. While there are many reasons for this, ensuring the documentation of important patient information so it appears accurately and appropriately in the patient record and is available to everyone on the health care team remains a top priority.

In an acute care environment, you will find that most of the coaching work takes place during the implementation of a new system or during a significant upgrade of an existing system. Important functions are moving into the electronic environment and need provider training and cooperation. One function is medication reconciliation. The Joint Commission and CMS mandate that a provider (not the nurse) account for all the medications the patient was taking upon admission, as well as the prescribed medication from the patient's hospital stay, and write new medication instructions that are clear, concise, and appropriate to their course of care. **Medication reconciliation (Med Rec)** is performed at the same time as the discharge orders and it is a tedious and sometimes frustrating process, depending on the system and software.

The outpatient environment provides many one-on-one opportunities to assist physicians in their use of EMR technology and is likely to be less intense. It is also spread out over a longer period of time as you work in close quarters with providers on a daily basis and can learn how and when to coach and when physicians are okay on their own.

In the outpatient setting, the use of **ePrescribing** software, which allows the provider to order a prescription for a patient and have it sent electronically to the patient's pharmacy, is an area most physicians want to master right away. There is high provider satisfaction reported for ePrescribing functions in the EMR. Other functions may not be as pleasing to the new adoptee of technology. Training a physician to use dropdown menus and a template instead of writing free text as they document patient care is a major culture and process change. Although many physicians are quickly adapting, other providers are slow to embrace the transition. Avoid preaching about the benefits of EMR data collection and be sympathetic to their frustrations. Learn how to read each individual to tailor your teaching and provide suggestions to best meet his needs for documentation compliance and greater efficiency.

As an EHR specialist, you can provide valuable coaching on the use and functionality of new and emerging software. For example, digital voice recognition is available as an option in many EMR applications for the physician office setting. This allows a physician to manage tasks he once paid others to complete. In the past, physicians dictated into a recording device and then sent it off for transcription by in-house transcriptionists, external transcription companies, or the office manager. While transcriptionists are not obsolete, they are fewer in number. Medical editors, however, are on the increase. Your support will help a physician in his adoption of **health information technology**, so he can better serve his patients.

Provide End-user Technical Support of EHR Software

With the implementation of certification requirements and the decrease of homegrown EHR and EMR solutions, technology support functions will likely fall to the professional IT department in larger facilities and hospitals or to the technology support team assigned to the physician office or clinic that was negotiated at the time of purchase or lease. In either case, it is a good idea for you, as an EHR specialist, to become as skilled as possible on the facility's system and to make connections with the vendor support department and team to minimize downtime and frustration in the department or facility.

Knowing whom to call and recognizing when to call before a major disaster wreaks havoc on the day is an important role for the EHR specialist.

Edit Existing Searchable Databases

Maintaining up-to-date patient information is critical in every health care setting. Your skills in managing data and information in the online environment helps the facility's data remain as accurate as possible in real time.

The process at many facilities for verifying patient information is to provide a form and a clipboard at patient check-in and ask the patient to complete the information. In computerized environments, some facilities print out a patient information page from the patient database and hand the patient a red pen, asking them to mark each portion as correct, or to edit incorrect data. This process differs little from previous decades. Enter the updated information into the appropriate **database** and the correct data prints from the patient's record at his next scheduled visit.

EHRs are complex, relational databases. Managing these databases differs little from managing a generic database in any other industry with one major exception: the information contained within many of the data tables is private, confidential, and protected by both federal and state law.

The first rule concerning the management of database information is the assignment of access privileges. In the hospital setting, this is a major undertaking. It's managed by the IT department in consultation with privacy and security professionals. In the smaller health care setting, the office manager may charge you with setting up access controls and privileges.

Role-Based Access Controls (**RBACs**) manage each person's access to specific areas in the information system. In a hospital setting, for example, a patient registration technician can only enter data specific to demographics, insurance information, and next of kin. The patient registration technician is not able to log in to see what procedures the patient underwent during the last admission, the laboratory values for the preoperative testing, or the results from a chest x-ray completed last month. The patient registration technician does not need this information to process the business side of the patient's admission. Similarly, a laboratory technologist does not need to view a patient's progress notes, so the RBAC system restricts her access to laboratory and related necessary tasks only. For a pharmacy example, a pharmacist can order medication within her scope of practice as defined by state law, but a pharmacy technician can only acknowledge and prepare a prescription for dispensing. RBACs are an important component of patient safety, as well as the protection of patients' private health information.

Regardless of the care setting, nonclinical personnel, which would be you, should not edit clinical areas of the patient record. You cannot edit progress notes or enter clinical data either unless your role expands to include tasks of a medical assistant or other clinical staff member.

Editing databases that house insurance company information, code sets, and other administrative information is important to maintaining up-to-date processes for the facility and remaining in compliance with the many legal and regulatory requirements for facilities. You may find this task as part of your job description. It is important to be aware of the time table for code set updates. The National Center for Health Statistics (NCHS) and CMS oversee the ICD-10-CM/PCS code updates, and when necessary, publish them twice a year, while the AMA annually reviews CPT codes. Insurance company information can change anytime. As the Affordable Care Act continues to impact health care, changes to insurance plans, new entrants to the market and mergers, acquisitions, and other business activities that relate to the health insurance industry will require you to remain up to date on this evolving industry and how it impacts patients.

Databases accessed remotely are generally not your responsibility to edit. However, if in the course of business you notice inconsistencies or errors, it is your professional duty to report them to the responsible party.

Identify Inconsistencies between Patient Information and Practice Management Software

In hospitals, larger facilities, and health systems, the implementation of an EHR system is a major undertaking that unfolds over a period of years after careful planning for the physical space, human resources, skill sets, and financial aspects. In addition, these installations involve major national firms with extensive experience in hospital information systems. Although this does not ensure there are never inconsistencies between patient data and the EHR software, it is less likely to occur in this environment. When it does occur, the likelihood is that the identification emerges from a clinical unit where a nursing or provider activity was unable to be captured. This report filters up through the EHR committee structure and lands at the appropriate desk where an HIM or IT professional handles the inquiry and resolves the issue.

In smaller facilities, such as providers' offices or clinics, you may discover that the preloaded EMR software is missing some aspect of practice the provider wants to use. Investigate the issue and return several resolution options to the clinical staff.

If the inconsistencies include missing terms from dropdown menus, this may only involve adding the terms to the database in the back end of the EMR software so they are available in the menu. If you get more complex requests, you may need to route them to the vendor or IT contracted professionals for assistance. People often credit super-computer capabilities to any computer in front of them. You will need to evaluate each request to determine whether there is an alternative, already-established path for the clinician to take, or if the task is being performed appropriately and the clinician is simply unhappy. In the latter instance, call the vendor or technology support line. Do not argue with the provider or other clinical staff person, even if you are sure about the answer. Putting distance and time between an aggravated physician and a technological problem, then calling in the experts is a much better option than getting into a contest of wills with someone who is already displeased with the situation.

It is also recommended for you to have a proactive approach to anticipated inconsistencies. Once you are settled into your new position, develop a short, easy-to-complete survey or questionnaire to capture any concerns the clinical staff may have about the software and how it captures patient or clinical information. Communicate to find solutions to these problems. Although not every request can be fulfilled, you should identify yourself to colleagues as a professional and valued team member.

Summary

As an EHR specialist, you are an important health care team member who can provide critical skills to hospitals, clinics, and physician offices. You need to understand the basic patient record and the laws, regulations, and guidelines that dictate practice. You also need to possess the ability to work in diverse and fast-paced environments. As technology continues to impact the way patients seek health care services and providers deliver them, your work will grow in scope, practice, and importance.

Drill Questions

1. An EHR specialist should perform which of the following actions to protect the private patient information within an EHR?

   A. Leave the computer logged in at all times so it is easy to access patient information without delay.
   B. Give her login ID and password to a coworker in case he needs to get information from her computer when she is out sick.
   C. Turn in an unidentified USB drive that she found into the IT department for evaluation.
   D. Download external content only from websites she knows are safe.

2. Which of the following describes the impact on legacy systems when implementing an EHR system?

   A. Legacy systems are built to work with other health information technology solutions.
   B. The EHR replaces legacy systems upon installation.
   C. Legacy systems require an interface to communicate with EHR systems.
   D. Legacy systems and EHRs process different data and can coexist in the same facility without special accommodations.

3. Which of the following is considered an incomplete record?

   A. A signed H and P report that was complete 1 week before the patient was admitted
   B. A discharge summary the provider has not signed 45 days after discharge
   C. A patient record that is partially paper and partially electronic
   D. A patient record that is missing important patient demographic or insurance data

4. Which of the following is the appropriate way for a provider to order physical therapy services for a patient in a hospital setting?

   A. ePrescribing
   B. eFax
   C. HIS
   D. CPOE

5. In a provider's office, which of the following helps providers document vaccines and immunizations safely and accurately?

   A. Clinical vocabularies
   B. Online references
   C. Clinical templates
   D. Barcode scanner

6. To participate in the financial incentive programs from the U.S. government, hospitals and providers must use an EHR or EMR system that is certified by which of the following?

   A. CMS
   B. NPDB
   C. CCHIT
   D. Joint Commission

7. A patient record that exists partially in a traditional, paper-based format and partially in a health information system is called which of the following?

   A. Hybrid record
   B. Incomplete record
   C. Continuity of care record
   D. Archived record

8. According to HIPAA regulations for the release of PHI, a hospital can release patient information in which of the following scenarios?

   A. A patient's wife requests the patient's record for insurance purposes
   B. A lawyer's office calls to request a review of the patient's record
   C. An insurance company requests a review of the patient's record to support the reimbursement request
   D. The HIM department has a ROI authorization on file for the patient relating to a previous admission

9. Which of the following restricts access to areas of the patient record or information system based on job title?

   A. CoPs
   B. RBACs
   C. EMR
   D. HIS

Drill Answers

1. An EHR specialist should perform which of the following actions to protect the private patient information within an EHR?

   A. Leave the computer logged in at all times so it is easy to access patient information without delay.
   B. Give her login ID and password to a coworker in case he needs to get information from her computer when she is out sick.
   C. Turn in an unidentified USB drive that she found into the IT department for evaluation.
   D. Download external content only from websites she knows are safe.

   EHR specialists should never introduce unknown media, such as a USB drive, into the information system. They should always turn in anything they find to the IT department so they can scan it for safety and return it to the rightful owner. Computers should not be left logged in when unattended. EHR specialists should not share their login ID and password with anyone. Downloading external content is always a risk and should be avoided on information systems that contain patient data.

2. Which of the following describes the impact on legacy systems when implementing an EHR system?

   A. Legacy systems are built to work with other health information technology solutions.
   B. The EHR replaces legacy systems upon installation.
   C. Legacy systems require an interface to communicate with EHR systems.
   D. Legacy systems and EHRs process different data and can coexist in the same facility without special accommodations.

   Interface software facilitates the communication or passing of data across and between systems that were not built to communicate with each other. Legacy systems represent a combination of manufacturers, operating systems, and platforms. They were not built to work with other health information technology solutions. Therefore, they will need some modification to communicate with other health information technology solutions. When there are legacy systems, the EHR is configured to communicate with them – even when a total system install takes place. Legacy systems represent departments that include pharmacy, laboratory, and radiology among others. The data from these departments is necessary for the functionality of the EHR. Therefore, EHRs and legacy systems cannot coexist in the same facility without special accommodations.

3. Which of the following is considered an incomplete record?

    A. A signed H and P report that was complete 1 week before the patient was admitted
    B. A discharge summary the provider has not signed 45 days after discharge
    C. A patient record that is partially paper and partially electronic
    D. A patient record that is missing important patient demographic or insurance data

The Joint Commission and CMS require records to be complete within 30 days after patient discharge. An unsigned discharge summary renders the record incomplete. An H and P report may be up to 30 days old. A patient record that is partially paper and partially electronic is a hybrid record. Although the data is incomplete, this does not render the record as incomplete.

4. Which of the following is the appropriate way for a provider to order physical therapy services for a patient in a hospital setting?

    A. ePrescribing
    B. eFax
    C. HIS
    D. CPOE

CPOE allows a provider to order medications, diagnostic testing, rehabilitation, and other services for inpatients. ePrescribing is the tool providers use in the outpatient setting to send prescriptions to the patient's pharmacy. It replaces the paper prescription pad. eFax is a software application that allows EHR specialists to send a document from the computer to a fax machine. HIS refers to the sum total of all information systems that support operations in a facility.

5. In a provider's office, which of the following helps providers document vaccines and immunizations safely and accurately?

    A. Clinical vocabularies
    B. Online references
    C. Clinical templates
    D. Barcode scanner

Barcode technology captures the information from medication barcodes and transfers this data into the record. This prevents inaccurate recording of details, such as dose, lot number, or expiration date. Clinical vocabularies help standardize the way providers use health care terms in the patient record. Online references provide cost-effective and up-to-date solutions for providers who need external information, such as the Physician's Desk Reference. Clinical templates make it easier for providers to document, but the templates have no impact on the accuracy of the documentation. For example, a provider could read a label incorrectly and administer the medication, then document in the template that he administered it.

6. To participate in the financial incentive programs from the U.S. government, hospitals and providers must use an EHR or EMR system that is certified by which of the following?

    A. CMS
    B. NPDB
    C. CCHIT
    D. Joint Commission

CCHIT approves and certifies EHR technology and is the required standard for facilities and providers wanting to participate in the Meaningful Use incentive program. CMS, NPDB, and the Joint Commission do not certify EHR products.

7. A patient record that exists partially in a traditional, paper-based format and partially in a health information system is called which of the following?

    A. Hybrid record
    B. Incomplete record
    C. Continuity of care record
    D. Archived record

A hybrid record is a record that is partially paper and partially electronic. An incomplete record is a record that is missing specific items, such as a provider's signature. Continuity of care records were an early solution for sharing patient data across facilities. Archived records are inactive and are in storage.

8. According to HIPAA regulations for the release of PHI, a hospital can release patient information in which of the following scenarios?

    A. A patient's wife requests the patient's record for insurance purposes
    B. A lawyer's office calls to request a review of the patient's record
    C. An insurance company requests a review of the patient's record to support the reimbursement request
    D. The HIM department has a ROI authorization on file for the patient relating to a previous admission

Under HIPAA regulations, patient records can be released for the purpose of treatment, payment, or to support the daily operations of the facility. Family members do not have the right to access each other's record without authorization. An attorney needs a ROI authorization to review a patient's record, even if the patient is her client. ROI authorizations must be specific and are valid for a limited period of time.

9. Which of the following restricts access to areas of the patient record or information system based on job title?

   A. CoPs
   B. RBACs
   C. EMR
   D. HIS

   RBACs restrict access to areas within an information system and are assigned based on the needs of the employee's job. CoPs do not restrict access to information. An EMR cannot restrict access to itself. HIS cannot restrict access to itself.

Terms and Definitions

Affordable Care Act – Mandates comprehensive health insurance reform; some of the provisions of this law include prohibiting the denial of coverage based on pre-existing conditions, preventing insurance companies from rescinding coverage when someone gets sick, eliminating lifetime limits or caps on insurance coverage, appealing insurance company decisions, providing free preventive care, getting tough on health care fraud, and extending the amount of time parents can cover their adult children on their own insurance policies; many more provisions are in place today and more will roll out through 2014

American Recovery and Reinvestment Act of 2009 (ARRA) – Consists of three major goals: create and save jobs, spur economic activity and invest in long-term growth, and support accountability and transparency in recovery spending

Authorization – Required for any release of patient PHI; consists of specific elements that make it legal and appropriate to release information

Business associate – An organization or individual who provides specific services to a covered entity involving the use or disclosure of PHI; for example, an off-site storage company that houses EMR data

Centers for Medicare and Medicaid Services (CMS) – Federal agency charged with administration of the Medicare and Medicaid programs, as well as the Children's Health Insurance Program; operating division of the Department of Health and Human Service (HHS)

Certification Commission for Health Information Technology (CCHIT) – Established to evaluate and approve EHR and EMR systems; to participate in incentive programs for EHR adoption and use, facilities must use a certified EHR or EMR product

Computer on Wheels (COW) – Most often refers to a laptop computer that sits on a cart with wheels that can be rolled from patient room to patient room and facilitates real-time documentation or charting of patient care; often called COWs

Computerized Provider Order Entry (CPOE) – Allows providers to order prescription medication, including IV therapies, laboratory tests, imaging studies, rehabilitation services, dietary requirements in the inpatient environment

Conditions of Participation (CoPs) – Specific practices that CMS mandates for facilities to follow if they treat patients covered under Medicare or Medicaid; similar to the Joint Commission's accreditation requirements

Continuity of Care Document (CCD) – The widely-accepted and federally-mandated document for sharing patient health information across facilities; replaced the CCR and CDA, which were earlier attempts at addressing the continuity of patient care between facilities

Continuity of Care Record (CCR) – An early form of a document developed to make communication about patients' course of care available across facilities; CCD replaced it

Covered entities – Providers who transmit PHI in an electronic format, health plans, and health care clearinghouses

Credentialing – Process used to document a provider's education, licensure, and qualifications in order to allow for the assignment of privileges to practice in a hospital or health care system

Current Procedural Terminology (CPT) – A nomenclature or naming system the American Medical Association (AMA) publishes and maintains; allows providers to code for services provided and submit bills for reimbursement

Database – Organized collection of pieces of information or data; electronic version of file cabinets with folders and files; the term generally refers to data collected and stored in an electronic environment

Digitize – Transform information from a paper-based document into an electronic format; some systems use document scanning that includes Optical Character Recognition (OCR) capabilities, which transforms a scanned document from a static image to a searchable document

Discharge summary – Report written by the provider when a patient is being discharged from inpatient care; summarizes the patient's chief complaint or why they were admitted to the hospital, diagnostic test results and other findings, treatments administered and how the patient responded to them; outlines recommendations for continued care and follow up, as well as dietary, medication and activity instructions; the provider must sign the final copy in the record before the record can be marked complete

Electronic health record (EHR) – While this term is generic, its use denotes a system-wide record that involves inputs from many systems and is used across a diverse environment of care with multiple location; although not strictly defined as such, EHR often refers to the electronic records in a hospital or integrated health care delivery system

EHR technology – Refers to the conceptual EHR, including the basic structure, functionality, and expected outcomes users expect from any system identified as being an electronic health or medical records system

Electronic medical record (EMR) – Another generic term for a digitized medical record; this term has evolved to most often refer to the single, standalone records systems that providers' offices and other smaller outpatient settings use; the term EMR is most often used in reference to the electronic records used by providers in their private practice and outpatient settings; many EMRs can exchange data with larger hospital-based EHR systems through the use of a Continuity of Care Document (CCD)

ePrescribing – Functionality that allows providers to prescribe medications to patients and send the prescription to the patient's pharmacy where it will process and be ready for pick up when the patient arrives; similar to CPOE from the inpatient environment in that clinical checking and alerts provide important safety measures for protecting patients

Fully-integrated EHR – Functionality that has replaced paper records entirely; few hospitals or health care systems in the U.S. have achieved this yet, but many are moving in this direction

Health Information Management (HIM) department – Department responsible for the care and management of all patient information; as electronic records began to replace paper-based records, HIM professionals became key players in the transition to the EHR or EMR system; previously known as the medical records department

Health information technology – General use of computers and related devices to manage the day-to-day functions in a health care environment

Health Insurance Portability and Accountability Act of 1996 (HIPAA) – Legislation that protects employees' insurance coverage when they are between jobs; people today are more familiar with what was formerly called Title II, or the Administrative Simplification provisions of HIPAA; Title II established national standards that apply to electronic transactions involving health care data and it is best known for addressing security and privacy protections for health care information

HIPAA Privacy Rule – Mandates the protection of patients' personal health information by hospitals and health care facilities, known as covered entities; provides a number of rights to patients in regard to their health information, but acknowledges there are times when disclosure of that health information is necessary for the provision of patient care and other business-specific purposes

HIPAA Security Rule – Sets forth the administrative, physical, and technical safeguards for covered entities in order to protect the confidentiality, integrity, and availability of PHI that is stored electronically

History and Physical (H and P) – Providers document a patient's history and perform a physical exam when she presents for health care services; this report is required to be filed in the inpatient record within 24 hr of admission for inpatients and cannot be more than 30 days old; this is often a dictated and transcribed report that must be signed by the physician before the record is considered complete

Health Information Technology for Economic and Clinical Health (HITECH) Act – Encourages the adoption and meaningful use of health information technology; has strengthened portions of the HIPAA Privacy and Security regulations to more aggressively protect patients' health information in the electronic environment; under this act, individuals and facilities that breach PHI are subject to harsher civil and criminal penalties

Hospital Information System (HIS) – Collection of systems that collect, store, and allow manipulation and management of data generated in the daily operations of a facility

International Classification of Diseases, 10th Revision, Clinical Modification (ICD-10-CM) – Coding and classification system that groups diseases and disorders into similar categories

Information Technology (IT) department – The IT department in facilities has emerged as a necessary response to the transition from a paper-based world to one that is increasingly reliant on technology for communications, data storage, management and retrieval, and delivery of patient care; those who work in the department work closely with all members of the health care delivery team to ensure patients' needs are met on every level

Joint Commission on the Accreditation of Health Care Organizations (The Joint Commission) – Not-for-profit and independent (non-governmental) organization that accredits and certifies more than 19,000 health care facilities and programs in the U.S.; accreditation from the Joint Commission is recognized nationally as the gold standard of accreditation and symbolizes the commitment to meeting high-quality standards in providing patient care

Legacy Information System – Department-specific systems that pre-date the implementation of EHRs by several decades; sometimes referred to as legacy systems

Master Patient Index (MPI) – Record of every patient who has been treated, seen, or evaluated in a facility; by law, this cannot be purged or destroyed after time and it must be forever maintained; also referred to as Master Patient/Person Index (MPPI)

Meaningful use – Meaningful use is both a program and a definition; the Meaningful Use program are the federal incentives established by CMS for facilities to use EHR technology in a meaningful way; meaningful use, the definition, refers to using EHR technology in a manner that makes a meaningful impact on patient care and safety

Medical Staff committee – A committee formed to discuss and recommend practices, policies, and other activities specific to the medical staff; this committee also oversees credentialing, or the assignment of privileges; in many hospitals, this committee reports to the Medical Executive Committee, which makes final decisions regarding the medical staff and is accountable to the board of directors and CEO

Medical terminology – The language of medicine, which encompasses terms to describe anatomy, physiological processes, disease, treatment, and other terms related to the human body and the care provided in terms of health and disease

Medication Reconciliation (Med Rec) – Process of gathering and documenting a complete list of a patient's medications when he is admitted to a care environment, which includes medications he was taking when he came into the facility and medications the provider prescribed as new and sending the list to the next care provider when the patient leaves the facility; CMS and the Joint Commission require participating facilities to perform medication reconciliation

National Practitioner Data Bank (NPDB) – A national database created in 1986 to collect information on licensed providers; providers are licensed by each state, and while bad behavior in one state can result in a loss of one's license to practice medicine, before the NPDB, bad providers were able to move to another state, seek licensure, and practice again

Off-site location – Off-site refers to remote or distant from the place of business; data recovery and storage options are often off-site, and many EMR solutions for providers exist in off-site locations and are accessed through a thin-client, or web portal; some hospitals also use off-site or remote access to EHR technology

Patient care orders (PCOs) – Patient interventions that are ordered by a provider for a nurse to carry out; these include guidance on how much assistance a patient needs to get out of bed; whether to document urinary output and liquid intake; medication orders that would not need approval by a provider each time, and dressing changes; also known as nursing orders

Physician's Desk Reference (PDR) – Traditionally this is a large, bound book that lists all prescription medications available on the market and includes prescribing information from the manufacturers; it is now available by subscription in an electronic format, accessible through EHR and EMR systems or though standalone electronic devices, such as a PDA or tablet PC

Protected health information (PHI) – Information that can individually identify a person; includes demographic data or any common identifier, such as Social Security number, date of birth, address, or phone number

Release of Information (ROI) – Appropriate and legal release of patient health information that includes PHI; HIPAA outlines the requirements for proper release of information in various circumstances

Role-Based Access Controls (RBACs) – Control the ability to access certain areas of the system, based on the person's role in the facility, which is associated with their login ID and password

Systematized Nomenclature of Medicine - Clinical Terms (SNOMED-CT) – A medical reference vocabulary that serves to standardize the naming of terminology used in medicine and health care

Templates – Pre-designed forms for the capture of data and information; common attributes of templates include dropdown menus, check boxes, and required fields, which will not allow the user to advance without answering the question or providing the data

Wireless on Wheels (WOW) – WOWs are the same as COWs; in some environments, patients may be sensitive to the casual use of the word cow, so some facilities prefer to use the WOW acronym to avoid any patient misunderstanding

02 INSURANCE AND BILLING

Learning Objectives

After reading this chapter, you will be able to:

- *Enter coding and billing information in the EHR.*
- *Abstract diagnoses and procedural descriptions from the medical record.*
- *Enter diagnoses and procedural descriptions from the medical record into the EHR.*
- *Generate insurance verification reports.*
- *Generate patient statements.*
- *Post payments to patient accounts at the time of visit.*
- *Generate encounter forms/superbills.*
- *Generate face/admission sheets.*
- *Find codes in the ICD*, CPT, and HCPCS manuals.*

Introduction

Patients who receive care from providers pay fees that support continuing operations of the facility. A patient may pay for medical services directly, called private or self-pay, or by using insurance.

In general, insurance pays for provider visits, laboratory and radiology tests, emergency department visits, hospitalization or inpatient services, outpatient services, and prescription medications. Insurance policies differ in the services they cover, deductible and copayment amounts, treatment options, and insurance limit amounts. An individual can purchase insurance directly from an insurance company or through an employer as part of a group plan. The U.S. government offers an insurance program called Medicare, which is available to individuals 65 and older and to people who have certain disabilities. Each state offers an insurance program called Medicaid, which covers patients who meet certain eligibility criteria and who are otherwise uninsured. Medicaid eligibility and coverage differs in each state so it is best to learn the guidelines for the state in which you work.

EHR software is a vital part of the health care industry. As an EHR specialist, you use insurance information to generate **insurance verification** reports, and you enter information you receive from the patient to generate the patient **face sheet**, which is also called an admission report or intake form. Then, you record payments made to the facility into the patient account.

In the electronic records environment, providers enter information directly into the EHR system at the point of care. Traditionally, coders take this information and assign a numeric code set to the encounter for the diagnosis and the procedure. However, in today's EMR software, many systems map ICD-10-CM/PCS and CPT codes to the menu items providers may choose during treatment that assigns the code when they document patient care. This enables the EHR specialist to verify the accuracy of the code assignment and to process the insurance claim and patient bill quickly and efficiently.

EHR technology allows for more streamlined documentation of patient care. This in turn enables providers to bill accurately, which supports an efficient revenue cycle that maintains financial stability for the facility.

Enter Coding and Billing Information in the EHR

In the health care setting, coding and billing provide the means for reimbursement to providers and facilities for their services. Therefore, these are extremely important steps in the health care workflow.

Medical codes come in various forms and evolved from different needs of the medical facility. The International Classification of Disease (ICD) is a classification and coding system that is in place around the world. In the U.S., ICD-10-CM/PCS is an integral part of the revenue cycle for hospitals and health care facilities.

ICD-10-CM captures diagnoses for inpatient and outpatient settings. ICD-10-CM disease and injury codes contain up to seven alphanumeric characters, such as T82.120S (Displacement of cardiac electrode, sequela). Assignment requires the interpretation of coding conventions (e.g., Code also, Excludes 1). The first character of an ICD-10-CM code is always a letter, and codes that contain four or more characters require the use of a decimal. The placeholder "x" is used when a seventh character is required but there is no fifth and/or sixth character, such as T14.8xxA (Other injury of unspecified body region, initial encounter).

ICD-10-CM contains an (1) Index to Diseases and Injuries, which includes a Neoplasm Table, Table of Drugs and Chemicals, and an Index to External Causes; and a (2) Tabular List of Diseases and Injuries. Main terms in the index are boldfaced, and subterms are indented. When using the ICD-10-CM index to locate a code, the tabular list must be reviewed to validate accuracy of code assignment.

In the inpatient setting, you will code procedures using ICD-10-PCS. ICD-10-PCS procedure codes contain seven alphanumeric characters (using letters A-H, J-N, and P-Z), such as 0DTJ0ZZ (Resection of Appendix, Open Approach). No decimal is used in ICD-10-PCS codes, and letters I and O are not used (because they could be confused with numbers 1 and 0). ICD-10-PCS contains an (1) Index and (2) Tables. Main terms in the index are boldfaced, and subterms are indented. When using the ICD-10-PCS index to locate a procedure, the appropriate table must be used to "build a code" (e.g., index main term "Appendectomy" directs the coder to table 0DTJ to locate the fifth through seventh characters, resulting in 0DTJ0ZZ for an open approach or 0DTJ4ZZ for a percutaneous endoscopic approach).

ICD-10-PCS procedures are organized into 17 sections, which include: 0 Medical and Surgical, 1 Obstetrics, 2 Placement, 3 Administration, 4 Measurement and Monitoring, 5 Extracorporeal or Systemic Assistance and Performance, 6 Extracorporeal or Systemic Therapies, 7 Osteopathic, 8 Other Procedures, 9 Chiropractic, B Imaging, C Nuclear Medicine, D Radiation Therapy, F Physical Rehabilitation and Diagnostic Audiology, G Mental Health, H Substance Abuse Treatment, X New Technology. The first character of an ICD-10-PCS code always corresponds to the section where the procedure is classified. The second through seventh characters have specific meanings, which are unique to each section.

In the outpatient setting or to capture procedures done by providers for their billing purposes, you should use the CPT code set. CPT codes capture medical, surgical, and diagnostic services providers perform and also are known as Level I HCPCS codes. **Healthcare Common Procedural Coding System (HCPCS)** consists of two levels. CPT codes make up Level I, while Level II codes capture services, supplies, and equipment for which no Level I or CPT code exists. An example of a HCPCS Level II code is A6412, which is an occlusive eye patch. If a patient receives this at an office visit, you should submit this HCPCS code to the insurance company for the payment of this item, in addition to the codes that represent the provider services and any other treatment or equipment.

Correct coding takes study, practice, and a commitment to staying up-to-date as the technology and profession evolves. As an EHR specialist, your role in coding and billing will vary depending on your place of employment.

Abstract Diagnoses and Procedural Descriptions from the Medical Record

Coding begins with the review of the documentation of patient treatment and course of care in the medical record. In the inpatient setting, coding is built off the principal diagnosis or reasons for admission. In the outpatient setting, the term principal diagnosis is not valid. Instead, you will look for the "first-listed diagnosis" to code outpatient visits.

To find the first-listed diagnosis, review the documentation from the patient visit. For the provider's office setting, review the provider's notes. This often presents in a format like this:

> "25-year-old female, established patient, presenting with painful urination, visible blood in urine. Urinalysis confirms presence of bacteria, nitrites. Urinary tract infection; prescribed Nitrofurantoin 100 mg, BID. Return to clinic in 2 weeks for follow up."

In this record entry, the diagnosis is clear: a urinary tract infection. The coding process for this patient would include the Evaluation and Management (E&M) code to capture the time spent by the clinician, and the ICD-10-CM diagnosis code. This patient underwent no procedures.

If the patient was in for a less specific issue that could not be identified without further testing, you would code the symptoms. Here is an example:

> "25-year-old male, established patient, presenting with pain in lower back. Reports moving heavy furniture previous week. Imaging studies ordered for lower back; patient prescribed rest, ice to affected area, and Flexeril 10 mg, TID. Return to clinic in 1 week for follow up."

In this record entry, there is no obvious diagnosis other than pain in the patient's lower back. Therefore, the code assignment would include the E&M code to capture the time spent by the clinician, and the ICD-10-CM diagnosis code for lower back pain only. This patient underwent no procedures.

As the examples above illustrate, knowing the medical record and the location of the various provider documentation sources is critical for accurate coding and appropriate reimbursement. Each EMR system will be set up uniquely to meet the needs of each facility. Understanding how providers document and where the information resides within the EHR system will make your job much easier.

Enter Diagnoses and Procedural Descriptions from the Medical Record into the EHR

Today, most coders use what is known as an encoder, which is software that helps assign codes for diagnoses and procedures. Encoders guide you in the assignment of codes, and in many cases, eliminate the need to search through hundreds of pages of books to locate a code.

Most EHR and EMR systems in use today come with an integrated encoding system or the ability to interface with an existing encoder. Some of these may already exist within the separate **practice management system**. Practice management software helps outpatient settings coordinate the business aspects of the office, such as appointments, insurance verification, and billing.

With the transition from paper forms to point-of-care documentation, many traditional workflows, such as coding from the paper encounter form, abstracting additional codes from the provider's notes, and other tasks, will change. Depending on your EMR software and the options it includes, providers may code patient encounters at the point of care as they are documenting. This is possible by using dropdown menus in the EMR clinical templates. If this is the case in your facility, your role in coding may be code editing rather than coding. Your responsibility would include reviewing the assigned codes for accuracy and verifying the documentation in the record supports the code assignment. Take advantage of as much continuing education as possible, either from your facility or the vendors of the practice management and EMR software, to help stay on top of the shifting workflows for coders, EHR specialists, and others.

Generate Insurance Verification Reports

The federal government's push for hospitals and providers at every level to move from paper-based to electronic records is producing more efficiency in the health care delivery system. One of those efficiencies is the payer portal, or the web-based access point facilities can use to verify insurance coverage quickly and accurately.

Many of the systems in place today can link to your patient scheduling system and allow you to upload information about patients in a batch to verify the status of each patient's coverage. This batch processing is much more efficient than entering each patient individually. However, most portals also provide verification on a patient-by-patient basis. They also can provide pertinent details, such as copayment or an estimate of the patient's expected contribution per visit type.

Reports for finance or other purposes may be part of the package your facility purchases when subscribing to a payer portal. If not, you may need to save batch data in spreadsheet software and create monthly, quarterly, annual, and ad hoc reports. This will vary by facility. Hospitals and larger clinics likely will have a process that involves regular reporting and is done in a finance or revenue cycle department. As an EHR specialist, your role in verifying insurance likely will focus on smaller outpatient clinic or provider's office settings where you assist in the entire patient business process, from registration to revenue receipt.

Generate Patient Statements

Health care facilities are businesses. When customers visit a retail store to purchase goods or services, they receive an invoice at the end of the transaction that highlights the items they are purchasing, as well as their method of payment. When patients present to a facility for health services, a detailed record captures the services, supplies, and other goods they received, along with the method of payment. In health care, the payment is most often some form of health insurance.

Electronic systems, such as practice management systems and EMRs, enable the quick processing of statements. Patient demographic data is collected and stored for multiple uses and combined with current information about the services accessed for a specific date. Prepare patient statements in layman's terms so patients can easily interpret what they are paying for and why.

Each facility's software configuration will affect the look and organization of the patient statement, but in general, statements should contain the following:

- Patient name

- Patient address

- Facility name, address, phone number, fax number, and website (where applicable)

- Patient insurance information

- Description of all services provided during the encounter

- Charges per service

- Date of services

- Provider name and **national provider identifier (NPI) number**

- Charges paid by insurance

- Charges due from the patient

Some statements will separate the specifics like diagnosis and procedures codes from the patient statements because they have little meaning to patients.

Depending on the software in use and the workflow in your facility, you may actively process patient statements each month or simply coordinate them from a **third-party vendor** or billing company that processes all of the facility's financial activity and records.

Post Payments to Patient Accounts at the Time of Visit

EHRs do not capture patient finance information. They do in many cases link with existing practice management systems or include modules that accommodate billing activity. Depending on the assignments in your facility, your role as an EHR specialist may include posting copayments or other forms of payment to patient accounts. In most practice settings, the patient must present an insurance card at the time of visit for verification. At this time, you also will collect any copayment, coinsurance, or other charges. Each facility should have a written financial policy in place that defines the procedures for collecting fees. This policy should outline the process for collecting copayments and identify which forms of payment, such as cash, credit card, or check, are acceptable. The policy should also cover the method of paying for services insurance companies do not cover, indicate when patients need to prepay for services, and determine if sliding-scale payments are an option.

Facilities will also maintain records for each day's patients to track all payments. These payments may be posted to patient accounts in real time or collected and entered later. With the widespread use of technology, many facilities post in real time. This process varies by facility, but the day sheet in some form is consistent across facilities, and is an integral part of the internal audit system.

Make certain to provide the patient with a receipt for any payments made, and do not generate statements until payments post in the system and are applied to the account.

Generate Encounter Forms/Superbills

In the outpatient setting, **encounter forms** have traditionally been produced in triplicate, or three parts, that the provider uses to document the E&M code, as well as any prescribed medications and a diagnosis. In today's increasingly electronic environment, these forms and many others have made the transition to the computer.

As more providers use point of care documentation with a laptop or tablet PC, the electronic encounter form as a clinical template becomes a seamless part of the encounter. This technology is driven by dropdown menus and pre-populated lists that enable quick entry into a form. They also allow the staff to expedite the patient check-out process, as well as the coding and bill generation.

EHR specialists may work to ensure all patient demographic information is accurate in the practice management and EMR systems, and then process the encounter forms after the patient exits the exam room. Once the encounter form is complete, the information can populate a superbill, or itemized bill for services. Depending on the level of integration and automation between the EMR and practice management system, your role may be minimal or may require attention to the details on the form and other documentation to generate the superbill. Each facility will have a specific process and workflow that meets the needs of patients, providers, and staff.

Generate Face/Admission Sheets

When a patient first enters a new health care system, the facility registers the patient by obtaining information and creating an account of the patient's identity and medical condition. The staff member who registers the patient will accurately identify the patient by complete name, date of birth, and Social Security number. As the registration clerk or other staff member enters the patient information into the software, the necessary information populates the face sheet, along with other areas in the information system.

A face sheet, also known as an admission sheet or intake form, is one or two pages that lists the patient's name, record number, date of birth, age, gender, religious preference, address, next of kin, Social Security number, insurance information, allergies, date of service, medical diagnosis, provisional diagnosis (if the provider has not seen the patient to confirm a diagnosis), chronic medical conditions, and selection of advance directives. The face sheet is always the first page of the paper medical chart. Each facility uses face sheets specific to the individual facility to better streamline its information. Facilities use the face sheet information for billing, medical history, notifying next of kin in emergency situations, and patient demographics. The face sheet is prominent in the patient's medical chart because it contains the most relevant patient information in a concise, predictable format.

Find Codes in the ICD, CPT, and HCPCS Manuals

In the electronic record setting, the practice of coding from book manuals is largely obsolete. However, there will be times when you need to verify a system-generated code or investigate a questionable code assignment. In these cases, you will need to know how to use the various coding manuals.

The ICD-10-CM manual contains symbols and conventions. Conventions are formats and notations that incorporate standards. Conventions include symbols, punctuation marks, notations, and abbreviations that assist in coding. You can find the legend for the conventions at the beginning of the manual. Each manual differs slightly by publisher. For accurate coding practices, EHR specialists and coders should be well-versed in symbols and conventions. Carefully note nonessential modifiers, code first notations, and primary or secondary coding notations.

CPT codes standardize accepted medical procedures and services into a numeric code for billing purposes. The numeric coding system creates a standard language to help the providers, insurance companies, and facilities communicate about patient care services. The AMA developed and maintains the coding system. Home health care agencies, providers' offices, hospices, assisted living facilities, birthing centers, nursing facilities, outpatient hospital services, and clinics use CPT codes.

The CPT manual contains three categories.

- Category I codes – Procedure and services codes, identified by descriptor nomenclature and the 5-digit CPT code. Category I codes are organized into six sections.

    - E&M

    - Anesthesia

    - Surgery

    - Radiology

    - Pathology and Laboratory

    - Medicine

- Category II codes – Optional use codes that track performance. These codes have four numbers followed by a letter, such as 1234A.

- Category III codes – Temporary codes for new technology. Category III codes have four numbers followed by the letter "T." After 5 years, these codes will be placed into the Category I codes area or removed from the CPT manual, depending on the usefulness of the codes.

The Category I area is divided into six sections that are further divided into subsections, categories, and subcategories. At the beginning of each section, specific guidelines further explain coding in the area and clarify codes.

The CPT manual contains 14 appendixes, labeled A through N, several of which the coder will use often. However, coders only use some appendixes in limited coding circumstances. A coder uses appendix A because it contains the modifiers needed to accurately code from the CPT manual. Appendix B lists CPT additions, deletions, and revisions. Coders use these to update encounter forms. Appendix D contains add-on codes, which define procedures and are never used as standalone codes.

Thoroughly read the guidelines at the beginning of each section and understand them before you begin coding the services. You should also always review the descriptions in all of the possible codes for a service before assigning a final code. You should always pay close attention to the place of service, such as a provider's office or nursing home because it affects which code to select. You should also pay close attention to the type of service provided, such as initial hospital care, subsequent hospital care, and consultation because this alters which code to select. Whenever you use an unlisted service code, submit supporting documentation to the insurance company, such as an explanation of what service the provider performed, pertinent findings, patient diagnosis, medical necessity of procedure or service, diagnostic or laboratory test findings, length of time of procedure or service, equipment needed for procedure or service, and follow-up care. The information you submit with the claim is linked directly to the revenue the facility receives. The more detailed the information, the better chance of cost recovery. There are some insurance companies that require HCPCS Level II national codes if the CPT manual does not contain the code for the service or procedure performed. Be sure to check the insurance company's rules before coding.

When you use computer-generated claim forms, the order you enter codes is important. When a provider performs multiple surgeries during the same period of time, rank them from major to minor. Insurance companies pay for the first procedure in full and the following procedures at a lower rate, usually from 50% to 75%. In the electronic environment it is easy to become complacent, but EHR specialists must monitor the computer-generated claim form to make sure the codes are accurately listed and sequenced for maximum reimbursement.

CMS created the National Correct Coding Initiative (NCCI) to assist in control of incorrect coding billed to Medicare and to assist in correct coding methods. NCCI edits are for providers' offices and outpatient services. NCCI recommends using Outpatient Code Editor (OCE) software for outpatient services and procedures that require bundled codes so the codes are reported correctly to avoid fraud. NCCI software offers several types of coding software for providers' offices. Under Medicare guidelines, claims denied under NCCI edits cannot be billed to the patient. Therefore, providers lose their reimbursement.

CMS developed the HCPCS coding system, which contains two levels.

- HCPCS Level I – CPT codes

- HCPCS Level II – Medicare's national codes

The CPT manual contains the majority of codes you need for patient procedures and services, but it is missing other patient care services. HCPCS Level II includes codes for durable medical equipment, orthotics, prosthetics, and other supplies and services. HCPCS codes can report services provided by providers, ambulance services, durable medical equipment companies, and non-physician providers, such as nurse practitioners and midwifes. HCPCS codes begin with a letter, A through V, and four numbers follow. If a code you need does not exist in the CPT manual, use the HCPCS code. Even though you use HCPCS codes for claims and billing, these codes do not guarantee service coverage. There are five types of HCPCS Level II codes.

- Permanent national codes

- Dental codes

- Miscellaneous codes

- Temporary codes

- Modifiers

Permanent national codes are alphanumeric codes for services and procedures. The HCPCS National Panel is the governing body that maintains the permanent national codes. The HCPCS National Panel is composed of representatives from the commercial health insurance, trade organizations, America's Health Insurance Plans (AHIP), CMS, and Blue Cross Blue Shield. All of these entities must agree before any changes to the permanent national codes can occur.

The American Dental Association (ADA) publishes codes for all dental procedures and supplies.

Use miscellaneous codes for products or services in which there is no pre-existing code. Claims for these codes must contain a complete description of the product or service, an explanation of why the patient needs the product or service, and information concerning the price of the product or service. Miscellaneous codes allow providers to bill products and services the Food and Drug Administration (FDA) recently approved. The HCPCS National Panel maintains temporary codes as a stop-gap measure to allow billing and payment for services that are not covered in the current permanent national codes. HCPCS members meet annually and discuss these temporary codes. If the members agree, the temporary codes are included in the next version of permanent national codes.

Modifiers are used with HCPCS Level II codes to clarify services and procedures providers perform on patients. Modifiers are two-character alphanumeric or alphabetic codes. HCPCS Level II codes are considered public domain and may be found on the CMS website.

Summary

The insurance and billing process is complex. The entire health care team works to properly document every patient encounter. This helps patients to receive the best care and facilities to capture revenue. EHR software assists facilities in streamlining the process of documenting patient care and billing for services. When the patient contacts the facility, the facility must obtain his or her personal information to verify insurance information. The patient's insurance information can be verified via phone, fax, mail, or the Internet. The fastest way to verify insurance information is to use a payer portal online. During the insurance verification process, coverage is confirmed, as well as any coverage limitations. The copayment is the amount the patient needs to pay before seeing the provider. The face sheet contains the patient's demographic information, current medical condition, and chronic diseases. The staff uses the face sheet as a quick reference for patient information.

There are three coding manuals you can use for billing purposes. Use ICD-10-CM codes to code the patient's diagnosis or physical condition. A patient's diagnosis can be documented only when confirmed by a clinician. However, EHR specialists can use symptomatic coding for provisional codes to establish a record until the clinician assigns a confirmed diagnosis. If the patient's procedure or service codes are not listed on the superbill or encounter form, use the CPT manual to code the procedures or services the patient received. Use the HCPCS Level II coding manual to code for durable medical equipment, supplies, services, and prosthetics. Some codes appear in both the CPT and HCPCS manuals. In this case, the insurance company decides which code they want you to use. To accurately code, carefully read the medical record and examine the procedure or service the patient received. Revenue depends on accurate coding.

Drill Questions

1. The NCCI recommends using which of the following for correct coding?

   A. A system where providers double-check coders
   B. "Un-bundling" codes
   C. Spreadsheet software
   D. Outpatient code editor software

2. When performing a coding review prior to submitting a reimbursement claim, an EHR specialist sees a code entered on an encounter form. Which of the following should she check for prior to submitting the claim?

   A. Provider's signature
   B. Supporting documentation
   C. Additional service code
   D. Patient's H and P report

3. Which of the following is included in the CPT manual?

   A. Health conditions
   B. Procedures and services provided by providers
   C. Conditions of Participation
   D. List of insurance companies

4. Which of the following is a common process for insurance verification?

   A. Payer portal
   B. Third-party insurance vendor
   C. Billing clearinghouse
   D. Patient management system

5. When assigning an ICD-10-CM diagnosis code, which of the following is correct?

   A. Use of the ICD-10-PCS is required.
   B. Use of the tabular list is optional.
   C. Use of the alphabetic index and tabular list are required.
   D. Assigning additional codes from the tabular list is optional.

6. Which of the following most likely would be billed using an HCPCS Level II code?

    A. A leg brace given to a patient in an office visit
    B. Sutures given to a patient who has an eye laceration
    C. A hysterectomy performed on a patient who has uterine cancer
    D. A comprehensive, detailed office visit

7. When abstracting from an outpatient record to assign the ICD-10-CM code, which of the following should an EHR specialist look for?

    A. Medications that were administered
    B. Diagnostic statement documented
    C. Presence of a consultation or second opinion
    D. Prescriptions that were written for the patient

8. When documenting a patient's reason for visit, the physician assistant typed in "sinusitis, acute" with no other details. In the ICD-10-CM coding software, an EHR specialist notices there are several options for coding sinusitis. Which of the following codes should the EHR specialist assign?

    A. J01 (acute sinusitis)
    B. J01.1 (acute sinusitis, frontal)
    C. J01.80 (acute sinusitis, other)
    D. J01.90 (acute sinusitis, unspecified)

9. Which of the following is included in the ICD-10-CM manual?

    A. Medical supply codes
    B. Durable medical equipment codes
    C. Surgical procedure codes
    D. Disease and injury codes

Drill Answers

1. The NCCI recommends using which of the following for correct coding?

    A. A system where providers double-check coders
    B. "Un-bundling" codes
    C. Spreadsheet software
    D. Outpatient code editor software

    The NCCI recommends using outpatient code editor software to ensure accurate coding and timely reimbursement. The NCCI does not recommend a system where providers double-check coders. Bundling may be appropriate in some circumstances. Spreadsheet software is a tool that can help organize data.

2. When performing a coding review prior to submitting a reimbursement claim, an EHR specialist sees a code entered on an encounter form. Which of the following should she check for prior to submitting the claim?

    A. Provider's signature
    B. Supporting documentation
    C. Additional service code
    D. Patient's H and P report

    All claims for reimbursement must be verified by documentation in the record. Providers' signatures, service codes, and patients' H and P reports are important, but they are not specific to this issue.

3. Which of the following is included in the CPT manual?

    A. Health conditions
    B. Procedures and services provided by providers
    C. Conditions of Participation
    D. List of insurance companies

    The CPT manual is published each year by the AMA and lists the procedures and services performed by providers in inpatient and outpatient settings. Health conditions are generally thought of as diagnoses and are not found in the CPT manual. Conditions of Participation are standards set by CMS that facilities must meet to be reimbursed for treating Medicare and Medicaid patients. The CPT manual does not list insurance companies.

4. Which of the following is a common process for insurance verification?

   A. Payer portal
   B. Third-party insurance vendor
   C. Billing clearinghouse
   D. Patient management system

   Payer portals streamline the insurance verification process by providing a single access for providers to verify all patients' coverage. A third-party insurance vendor will not provide insurance verification beyond their services. A billing clearinghouse is a company that processes bills for providers. Practice management systems help facilities coordinate business practices, such as patient flow and billing.

5. When assigning an ICD-10-CM diagnosis code, which of the following is correct?

   A. Use of the ICD-10-PCS is required.
   B. Use of the tabular list is optional.
   C. **Use of the alphabetic index and tabular list are required.**
   D. Assigning additional codes from the tabular list is optional.

   Coding accuracy and guidelines require the use of both the alphabetic index and the tabular list. Each of these components of the ICD-10-CM coding manual may contain information or instructions that are not included in the other. A complete and accurate code assignment is made by reviewing codes located in the index and then verifying codes referenced in the tabular list.

6. Which of the following most likely would be billed using an HCPCS Level II code?

   A. A leg brace given to a patient in an office visit
   B. Sutures given to a patient who has an eye laceration
   C. A hysterectomy performed on a patient who has uterine cancer
   D. A comprehensive, detailed office visit

   HCPCS Level II codes capture outpatient goods and services that include durable medical equipment, such as orthopedic braces. Sutures performed by a provider would be captured with a CPT (Level I HCPCS) code. A hysterectomy performed on a patient with uterine cancer would be coded as an ICD-10-PCS procedure code in the hospital inpatient setting. A comprehensive, detailed office visit is billed using the E&M codes in the CPT manual.

7. When abstracting from an outpatient record to assign the ICD-10-CM code, which of the following should an EHR specialist look for?

    A. Medications that were administered
    B. **Diagnostic statement documented**
    C. Presence of a consultation or second opinion
    D. Prescriptions that were written for the patient

    In the outpatient or provider setting, the EHR specialist should code the diagnostic statement documented. ICD-10-CM does not classify medications. Although the presence of a consultation, second opinion, and prescriptions that were written for the patient are important, they are not relevant for assignment of the diagnosis code.

8. When documenting a patient's reason for visit, the physician assistant typed in "sinusitis, acute" with no other details. In the ICD-10-CM coding software, an EHR specialist notices there are several options for coding sinusitis. Which of the following codes should the EHR specialist assign?

    A. J01 (acute sinusitis)
    B. J01.1 (acute sinusitis, frontal)
    C. J01.80 (acute sinusitis, other)
    D. **J01.90 (acute sinusitis, unspecified)**

    Because there is no additional information provided in the documentation, the EHR specialist should assign the code J01.90 (acute sinusitis, unspecified). The EHR specialist should not assign codes that include additional details or specifications that are not included in the documentation. The EHR specialist should not use only the classification or 3-digit code when 4th or 5th digit codes are available.

9. Which of the following is included in the ICD-10-CM manual?

    A. Medical supply codes
    B. Durable medical equipment codes
    C. Surgical procedure codes
    D. **Disease and injury codes**

    The ICD-10-CM coding manual is used to assign disease and injury codes. Medical supplies and durable medical equipment codes can be found in the HCPCS Level II coding manual. The ICD-10-PCS coding manual contains codes for surgical procedures.

Terms and Definitions

Current Procedural Terminology (CPT) codes – Numeric codes developed by the American Medical Association (AMA) to standardize medical services and procedures

Encounter form – A form the provider fills out as she sees the patient; lists the service charges and how much the patient paid for the services; can be submitted for billing

Face sheet – A standard structured document that contains patient information, such as name, date of birth, insurance information, reason for seeking medical care, and religious preference; medical staff uses the document to quickly see the relevant points for patient care

Healthcare Common Procedure Coding System (HCPCS) – A numeric and alphabetic coding system used for billing and pricing of procedures, medical supplies, medications, and durable medical equipment

International Classification of Diseases, Tenth Revision, Clinical Modification (ICD-10-CM) codes – Coding and classification systems that group diseases, disorders, and procedures into standardized codes

Insurance verification – Process used to make sure the service received by the patient is approved and paid for by the insurance company

National provider identifier (NPI) number – A unique 10-digit number assigned to providers in the U.S. to identify themselves in all HIPAA transactions

Practice management system – A software designed to assist in the office workflow by streamlining scheduling, insurance information, patient demographics, and billing

Third-party vendor – A separate business that handles a specific task for a facility; common third-party vendors include billing companies, transcription companies, and coding firms

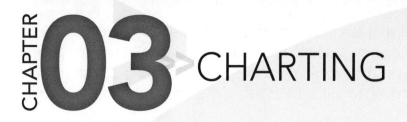

Learning Objectives

After reading this chapter, you will be able to:

- *Monitor provider documentation for completeness and accuracy.*

- *Categorize patient's health information into a reliable and organized system that promotes error identification.*

- *Enter live data into an EHR.*

- *Assist clinicians with charting.*

- *Locate requested information in a patient's chart.*

- *Execute file maintenance procedures, such as purging, archiving, finalizing, and securing.*

- *Audit charts to ensure compliance of proper charting.*

- *Document the link between effective charting and reimbursement for procedures clinicians perform.*

Introduction

The patient medical record in any form is the legal record of the care clinical staff members provide, the response the patient experiences to that care, and the eventual outcomes of that care. The record provides proof of high-quality care and care that falls short. It documents the professional decision making and provides an important historical record of what happens to patients in a variety of medical circumstances.

Helping the clinical staff appreciate the importance of accurate and complete charting is a job that never ends. When you assist providers in your facility to practice high-quality documentation, you contribute to better patient care. Precise documentation leads to fewer mistakes, better patient outcomes, a more stable **revenue cycle**, and better statistical data.

Monitor the Provider Documentation for Completeness and Accuracy

Complete and accurate documentation is the foundation of quality patient care and it supports appropriate reimbursement and revenue for the facility. The patient population needs pertinent documentation and that documentation needs to abide by the laws and regulations that govern health records. Each state has laws that dictate how long to keep each record, as well as policies on the acceptable methods for record destruction. In addition to state laws, facilities also need to abide by regulatory and government agency requirements for records.

Hospitals and health care facilities that treat Medicare or Medicaid patients are required to meet CoPs, which were developed by CMS. The goal of CoPs focuses on setting safety and health standards, which include improving the quality of care and protecting patients' health and safety. Facilities that fall under the jurisdiction of CMS include ambulatory surgical centers, outpatient rehabilitation facilities, critical access hospitals, end-stage renal disease facilities, home health agencies, hospices, hospitals, rural health clinics, and long-term care facilities.

Along with dictating important patient care provisions, such as requiring a hospital to have an adequate number of registered nurses, licensed practical nurses, and other personnel, CoPs specifies the content and management of health records. Each care environment has requirements that are specific to its patient populations. As an EHR specialist, familiarize yourself with the requirements that are relevant to your facility.

In hospitals, the CoPs for Medical Record Services require the establishment of a formal medical records, or health information management (HIM), department that is staffed by an appropriate administrator and makes patient records available to support patient care, while protecting the integrity and confidentiality of the records. CMS requires facilities to maintain records for at least 5 years. CoPs also specify the details necessary for a complete record. A complete record includes the patient's history and physical examination, admitting diagnosis, clinical evaluation results, documentation of complications, hospital-acquired infections, negative medication reactions, consent forms, orders, progress notes, treatment reports, medication records, reports from diagnostic testing, and documentation of patient information, such as vital signs. All of the information within the record assists providers in monitoring the patient throughout her hospital stay. Lastly, CMS requires each record to include a discharge summary, highlighting the patient's course of care and her response to the care. The record must also be complete, and the provider should authenticate all items by signing and dating all items in the record within 30 days of the patient's discharge.

As an EHR specialist, you may work in an HIM department and generate reports with data on these and other areas of interest from the EHR system. To assist providers in providing complete and accurate documentation in the patient record, it is important for you to know record components and the requirements for each. Before the implementation of electronic records, most HIM departments had a room dedicated to **incomplete charts.** Today's information systems streamline this process through the use of **database queries**, or reports. Queries guide the database to quickly search millions of records and return a report with details on which records are missing key items, such as a signature on the discharge summary, a history and physical report, or a dictated operative report.

Outpatient facility documentation standards differ from inpatient standards. They usually follow the guidelines the appropriate accreditation agency recommends. Accreditation for outpatient facilities is available through a handful of organizations, including the Joint Commission, the Accreditation Association for Ambulatory Health Care, and the Commission on the Accreditation of Rehabilitation Facilities (CARF), which accredits facilities that provide services to aging populations, behavioral health patients, and rehabilitation patients. Rehabilitation includes the dispensing of durable medical equipment, prosthetics, orthotics, and similar supplies. Some substance abuse treatment programs are also CARF-accredited. Larger clinics and ambulatory surgery centers may choose to seek out external accreditation, but providers' offices usually do not. Documentation practices remain consistent across care environments, regardless of accreditation status.

In an outpatient setting, you may need to set up special reporting from the EMR if it did not come pre-loaded in the software. If it is not already part of the practice management tasks, contact the EMR **vendor**'s technical support to learn about the feature the first time you attempt to set up special reporting. Once you identify documentation areas that are chronically problematic, such as a missing signature on a patient visit note, you can work with the clinical staff to pay closer attention to these areas and develop tools to assist them in remembering when and where to document.

Reimbursement, **compliance**, and quality patient care depend on proper documentation. Your role in monitoring the accuracy and completeness of patient records is an important part of patient care in your facility.

Categorize Patient's Health Information into a Reliable and Organized System

One of the major advantages to EHR systems is the structure they provide in the collection and organization of patient and related health data. In a traditional, paper-based medical record, there are ample opportunities to misfile data. Provider documentation can range from sparse to detailed.

In both inpatient and outpatient settings, the adoption and use of EHR technology improves the collection, organization, and availability of patient data.

EHR technology is not fool-proof. You cannot assume a paper record needs careful review, while the online system automatically corrects errors and does not also need a careful review. Be sure to learn the systems in your facility because it is an important part of supporting quality patient care.

The importance of quality documentation can be illustrated with the acronym **GIGO**, which stands for garbage in – garbage out. As an EHR specialist, it is your job to help the clinical staff enter complete, accurate, and error-free data during documentation to eliminate the garbage that causes incomplete records and errors, which may result in an inappropriate diagnosis, decreased reimbursement, or bad patient care documentation.

In a hospital or inpatient setting, the Medical Staff Executive Committee establishes documentation guidelines and codifies them, or makes them into rules. Medical Staff Bylaws provide rules the clinical staff must follow when documenting in patient records at the facility. While the bylaws may differ from facility to facility, they all follow standards put forth by CMS, and the Joint Commission where applicable, for the timely and accurate completion of the medical record. You may develop clinical templates and reminders in accordance with your facility's Medical Staff Bylaws.

In an outpatient or provider's office setting, standard practice for documentation is set by the physician owner or administrators in consultation with the providers, and abides by the standards necessary for compliance with regulatory agencies. As an EHR specialist, learn the system your facility uses, as well as the habits and needs of the clinical staff. This knowledge, along with your experience, makes you an important part of the health care team.

Enter Live Data into an EHR

You know now what you need to do to store patient data in an EHR. You also know that only clinical staff can legally document patient care in the record. However, you may enter patient demographic data, insurance information, or other nonclinical data.

In a hospital or larger clinic setting, your assignment may be in a business office or clerical environment, whereas in a provider's office, your work environment may be closer to the patient care areas. Depending on where you work, your tasks and the amount of contact you have with providers will vary.

The HITECH Act requires providers to use EHR technology in a meaningful way, which includes the use of templates and populated dropdown menus with point-and-scroll options for documenting patient care. Clinical templates guide clinician documentation and help prevent incomplete records. Reminders that trigger patient questions and require an answer in the electronic record are also useful. This technology enables providers to quickly and accurately enter information into a standard form. While it is necessary for providers to have a free text option to specify complex or unusual situations, you should use structured formats to store these findings as discrete or structured data. These findings should meet federal guidelines for meaningful use and support higher quality documentation. When you use structured data, it is easier to access information and to run a query.

When entering data, clinical or clerical, it is important to pay attention to details and focus on accuracy. Submitting an improper code for reimbursement may hold up payment for services, or worse – result in an audit for suspected fraud or abuse. Entering data hastily for a new patient can result in errors that misroute patient communication, insurance claims, or other important information.

Assist Clinicians with Charting

EHR specialists who work in an acute care setting rarely find opportunities to assist clinical staff in the day-to-day charting function. Assisting the clinical staff with day-to-day charting occurs in a concentrated period of time during a hospital-wide system implementation or major upgrade. You are more likely to provide charting assistance when you work in an outpatient or ambulatory care setting.

If you work in an outpatient environment, you will find you work much closer and more often with the clinical staff than you would in an acute or inpatient setting. This proximity provides you with the opportunity to observe clinical staff behaviors and note when they ask for help and which providers consistently have documentation errors or incomplete records. By using reports you run from the EMR, along with your observations and interactions, you can effectively assist providers with improving their documentation practices.

EHR technology is improving documentation by providing the opportunity for the clinical staff to chart as they provide patient care. **Point-of-care (POC) charting** or documentation reduces or eliminates the time between the provision of care and documenting in the record, which increases the likelihood the documentation is accurate, detailed, and complete.

In a hospital setting, the clinical staff accomplishes widespread POC charting through the use of COWs or WOWs. Many hospitals also give providers laptops or tablet PCs, so the EHR technology is more attractive and the documentation is easier to accomplish. Hospitals are using technological advancements to entice EHR adoption as one way to increase provider buy-in and compliance.

In the outpatient setting, busy clinical staff members are increasingly finding laptops and tablet PCs a convenience as they move quickly from patient to patient between examination rooms. As an EHR specialist, you can provide important support and training for clinical staff whose technology skills fall short and actively contribute to improving documentation in your facility and its patients.

Locate Requested Information in a Patient Chart

EHR specialists play an important role in communicating patient information to appropriate health record data users. Therefore, you must be familiar with the data and where it resides in the patient record or chart.

Fortunately, unlike paper-based records, almost all electronic systems include a search function, which allows you to navigate even a new system with little assistance. Most record search functions will likely involve you finding a specific patient in order to view data from his record. As with many computer tasks, there are several ways to find a patient. The best way to identify or locate a patient is to use the patient's medical record number (MRN). In small- to medium-sized practices, you could also elect to do a search by patient last name. If your search results return with too many patients to efficiently review, go back and add more criteria to the search, such as the patient's first initial of his first name. In hospitals or larger facilities, this may return a long list of patients. If adding additional name criteria is not helping to narrow the pool of results, try using a different data point, such as a patient's ID or home telephone number.

Once you locate the patient record you are searching for, find the results or other data you need. At this point in the search, there is no substitute for knowing the system. Standardization across EHR platforms is minimal – what is intuitive to find in one system can be hidden like buried treasure in another system. Spend time in the system you work with so you can quickly navigate to any area in the record with minimal hunting time.

Depending on the reason for locating the data, you will provide the information to the requesting clinician, patient, or other authorized party. Knowledge of the location of various data in the record is useful not only when you need to retrieve data to fulfill a request or to answer a clinician's question, but your skills to quickly navigate to the appropriate record location can assist the clinical staff in learning to quickly navigate and become independent users of the EMR.

Execute File Maintenance Procedures

State laws and other regulatory requirements dictate how long patient records should remain available. Each facility should consult legal counsel to determine the best course of action. Attorneys consider the patient population, whether it is pediatric, adult, general population, or specialty care, as well as applicable state and federal laws, when recommending a schedule for purging, archiving, or destroying inactive records.

Paper-based records present challenges to storage because of space limitations. Many record management businesses use vast underground storage areas that require golf carts to travel from one end to the other. However, paper records are easier to destroy than electronic records.

Electronic records take up less physical space than paper-based records, and archiving and retrieval of archived data is often simpler in electronic format. However, electronic records present a few challenges. One challenge is locating data that were once stored on an old computer drive. Another is destroying electronic media when record destruction is appropriate. As with paper-based facilities, facilities with electronic records must also have a **record retention** and a **record destruction policy** in place. One of the biggest challenges to electronic record destruction is keeping track of the places health information resides and appropriately disposing of equipment.

Facilities move at a fast pace, and computers that stop working are moved aside so working computers can replace them and business can proceed. Ideally, your facility policy should outline specific actions to take when a computer is no longer in active service. This includes not only deleting all files, but running a software utility to scrub the hard drive or using a magnetic erase function to corrupt the data. As portable technology continues to put protected patient information in more places, hospitals and health care facilities are challenged to manage and protect patient records.

When considering the storage of archive records, the issue is less of storing records and more of a data management consideration. Many options exist for the off-site storage of data, and weather-related disasters, such as tornadoes, floods, and hurricanes, highlight the importance of redundant data and off-site, or remote, storage options. For example, physicians in a midwestern town were back in business within 72 hr after a tornado destroyed the town because they used EHRs and off-site, **redundant**, or repetitive, **data storage**.

As an EHR specialist, your role in storing, archiving, purging, and destroying data may take many forms and may depend on the facility you are working in, the complexity of the information systems in place, and the laws and regulatory requirements in the state where you work.

Audit Charts to Ensure Compliance of Proper Charting

EHR software and information system technology make tasks from the paper-based world almost obsolete. Patient records, whether in an inpatient or an outpatient care setting, store volumes of data in different locations within the same record.

In facilities with an HIM department, the department handles all chart audit functions. As an EHR specialist, you may work in an HIM department, which means you may be the one who runs these reports. You will likely have a regular schedule to follow so you do not have to scramble at the end of every fiscal year or when a regulatory agency, such as CMS, or an accrediting agency, such as the Joint Commission, plans a visit. In the outpatient setting, your role as an EHR specialist may already include this task. If it does not, you may realize it is important and develop it for the facility. In inpatient or outpatient settings, the reporting capabilities within your facility's EHR solution allow you to run canned, or pre-loaded, reports or easily set up or program **ad hoc reports** to return the data you need after querying the records database.

In smaller or outpatient settings, reach out to your EMR vendor or your technical support contacts if you have questions about generating reports from within the EMR. This function is basic in the most rudimentary systems. The increasing requirements for EMRs to capture discrete, or structured data, makes it easier to query for the presence or absence of data points, thereby completing most audit reporting in a short period of time.

Document the Link between Effective Charting and Reimbursement

The process through which facilities receive payment for services they provide is known as the revenue cycle. The revenue cycle is a multi-step process that begins with providing services. After delivering services, whether in an inpatient or outpatient environment, the providers document the care in the patient record. From this documentation, the billing function establishes charges related to the documented care. This is called charge capture and refers to the documentation and capturing of all goods and services the facility or provider provides that generates a charge. In both inpatient and outpatient facilities, a database exists that is known as the charge description master (CDM), which is a list of each good and service patients can receive at the facility. The database lists items, such as vaccines, gauze dressings, or MRIs, along with a unique identification number or charge code, the department the item or service belongs to, such as radiology or central supply, the cost or price assigned to the item or service, a revenue code, and if applicable, the HCPCS code. In some facilities, there is also a column or field that denotes if the item is active or inactive. The CDM is the price list for anything a patient may use. When a patient bill is generated, the CDM is the source for assigning the cost of each line item. After that, the charge is applied to the patient bill.

Once the bill is complete, an internal review takes place. Many facilities use software called scrubbers, which are specific to individual payers, to check the claims for errors before submission. Some common oversight errors include invalid procedures, such as a hysterectomy on a male patient, incorrect service dates, or inappropriate code assignment. Facilities that do not use scrubbers perform audits by hand to ensure there are minimal claim rejections because of fixable mistakes. Once the claim is ready, the facility submits it to the appropriate third-party payer, and then the account moves into an accounts receivable status where the facility counts the claim as expected revenue.

When organizations submit claims for reimbursement to either public or private **payers**, HIPAA requires three code sets: ICD-10-CM, ICD-10-PCS, and HCPCS, and two categories of information: diagnosis codes and procedure/service codes. All providers, including hospitals and physicians, must use ICD-10-CM to report diagnoses. ICD-10-PCS is the code set HIPAA requires hospitals to use when reporting procedures on inpatients. HCPCS is the code set HIPAA requires for provider services and for hospitals to use when reporting outpatient services. It is important to remember that HCPCS Level I codes are CPT codes.

Accurate coding is important in both inpatient and outpatient settings. Coding has serious implications if performed incorrectly. For example, coding bronchitis as pneumonia is fraud and is punishable at the federal level, including fines and, in some cases, jail time. This is known as **upcoding** or maximizing. In the acute care or inpatient environment, the principal diagnosis drives the **diagnosis-related group (DRG)** assignment, which determines payment. Assigning a code that is not supported by the record documentation can result in major problems for you and your facility.

In an outpatient setting, an example of upcoding is submitting higher level E&M codes than the patient visit and documentation support. For example, the physician provides a problem-focused service, but assigns an E&M code for a detailed and comprehensive exam. Upcoding in the outpatient setting also happens by assigning a higher level diagnosis, such as coding a visit for chest pain due to anxiety as a heart patient work-up. Because there are criminal charges and fines associated with upcoding and fraud, many new or inexperienced coders code cautiously. Sometimes, this results in under-coding. As an EHR specialist, you can run a report to show the range of E&M codes assigned to determine accuracy and under-coding. Under-coding is not a crime, but it results in facilities receiving lower reimbursement than what they receive for the services they provide.

Providers' care and treatment of patients must appear in the chart accurately so the services they provide generate the appropriate reimbursement. EHR technology helps providers in all care settings document more precisely through the use of templates, flow sheets, dropdown menus, and other tools.

You can help the clinical staff in your facility better understand the link between accurate and complete documentation and reimbursement. You can also support them in achieving this through helpful reminders, EHR user support, periodic reviews, and reminders about documentation guidelines.

Summary

The patient record is the foundation for quality patient care, both in the short term and long term. It also provides solid documentation to support the revenue cycle, which is essential for facilities to remain in business. EHR specialists can contribute to quality patient care by supporting and monitoring clinical staff documentation and providing any assistance they may need in charting patient information.

Understanding the importance of basic file maintenance and performing these duties on a regular schedule supports best practices in maintaining information systems. You should also become an expert on the locations of the many data elements within the medical record so you can provide knowledgeable guidance to clinicians and others on the proper way to document important patient information. By ensuring that clinicians understands the proper way to document, it ensures the facility remains in compliance with the various legal and regulatory agency requirements that govern health records. Lastly, as an EHR specialist, you can learn the relationship between effective documentation and appropriate reimbursement and share the best practices for achieving this with your clinical staff and other colleagues.

Drill Questions

1. An EHR specialist has the medical record of a patient who was admitted through the emergency department and stayed in the hospital 7 days. The patient lives out of state and never returned to the facility after discharge. Which of the following applies to the patient's record?

   A. The record may not be destroyed unless the EHR specialist receives signed documentation from the patient stating he lives out of state and will never be back in the facility.
   B. The record may not be destroyed.
   C. The record may be destroyed after 5 years.
   D. The record may be destroyed based on the information collected from the patient at the time of treatment.

2. A facility has records on more than 500,000 patients, both past and present, in its EHR patient database. An EHR specialist needs to run a report that returns all of the patients one particular provider treated. The EHR specialist should use which of the following to obtain this report?

   A. Query
   B. Analysis
   C. Purge function
   D. Archive function

3. Which of the following is a form of charting that helps to improve documentation by having the provider document while they are with the patient?

   A. Problem-oriented
   B. At-the-elbow
   C. Patient-focused
   D. Point-of-care

4. Which of the following code sets is a provider required to include when submitting claims to public or private payers for reimbursement?

   A. ICD-0-3
   B. HCPCS
   C. SNOMED-CT
   D. LOINC

5. Which of the following qualifies as meaningful use of EHR technology?

  A. Using the computer to set patient appointments
  B. Using a prepared letter to provide patient referrals
  C. Using a clinical template to guide patient assessment
  D. Using the computer system to search the internet for diagnosis information

6. Reluctant adopters of EHR technology find which of the following beneficial?

  A. Clinical templates
  B. Point-of-care (POC) charting
  C. ePrescribing
  D. Online references

7. Storing data off-site in more than one location is referred to as which of the following?

  A. Duplication
  B. Redundancy
  C. Virtual storage
  D. Archival storage

8. When removing computer equipment from service that once contained PHI, which of the following is accepted as a guarantee for preventing a privacy breach?

  A. Deleting all files
  B. Running a software scrub utility
  C. Disassembling and recycling the computer parts
  D. Reusing the equipment as long as it remains in the original facility

9. A provider's office that routinely submits reimbursement claims for allergy-related coughing as chronic asthma may be committing which of the following?

  A. Plagiarism
  B. Upcoding
  C. Medical malpractice
  D. Coding malpractice

Drill Answers

1. An EHR specialist has the medical record of a patient who was admitted through the emergency department and stayed in the hospital 7 days. The patient lives out of state and never returned to the facility after discharge. Which of the following applies to the patient's record?

   A. The record may not be destroyed unless the EHR specialist receives signed documentation from the patient stating he lives out of state and will never be back in the facility.
   B. The record may not be destroyed.
   C. The record may be destroyed after 5 years.
   D. The record may be destroyed based on the information collected from the patient at the time of treatment.

   CMS allows for the destruction of health records after 5 years. However, state laws may have stricter or longer requirements and should be checked before any record is destroyed. Record retention and record destruction is bound by state and regulatory agency requirements.

2. A facility has records on more than 500,000 patients, both past and present, in its EHR patient database. An EHR specialist needs to run a report that returns all of the patients one particular provider treated. The EHR specialist should use which of the following to obtain this report?

   A. Query
   B. Analysis
   C. Purge function
   D. Archive function

   A query is used to pull records from a database based on specific criteria. An analysis is undertaken after the records are retrieved. The purge function removes data and records from a database. The archive function removes files from an active status and places them in storage or inactive status.

3. Which of the following is a form of charting that helps to improve documentation by having the provider document while they are with the patient?

    A. Problem-oriented
    B. At-the-elbow
    C. Patient-focused
    D. Point-of-care

Point-of-care documentation refers to the ability of EHR technology to provide quick, easy-to-navigate documentation tools that allow the provider to document as she is interacting with the patient. Problem-oriented charting refers to documentation in the record, not the approach. At-the-elbow refers to coaching the clinical staff in the adoption and use of EHR technology. A patient's exam should be patient-focused, as well as his documentation. However, it is not the form of charting the provider performs while she is with the patient.

4. Which of the following code sets is a provider required to include when submitting claims to public or private payers for reimbursement?

    A. ICD-0-3
    B. HCPCS
    C. SNOMED-CT
    D. LOINC

HIPAA mandates that providers submit reimbursement claims using HCPCS and ICD-10-CM/PCS code sets. ICD-0-3 is an oncology code set. SNOMED-CT codes are not used for reimbursement purposes. LOINC is a database and universal standard for identifying medical laboratory observations.

5. Which of the following qualifies as meaningful use of EHR technology?

    A. Using the computer to set patient appointments
    B. Using a prepared letter to provide patient referrals
    C. Using a clinical template to guide patient assessment
    D. Using the computer system to search the internet for diagnosis information

Using clinical templates when assessing patients meets the requirements for meaningful use. Using the computer to set patient appointments, using a prepared letter to provide patient referrals, and using the computer system to search the Internet for diagnosis information does not meet the requirements for meaningful use.

6. Reluctant adopters of EHR technology find which of the following beneficial?

    A. Clinical templates
    B. Point-of-care (POC) charting
    C. ePrescribing
    D. Online references

Reluctant adopters of EHR technology find ePrescribing useful and a positive addition. Some providers appreciate templates, while others prefer writing their own documentation notes. Some providers enjoy the convenience of POC charting, while others struggle to manage communicating with the patient and typing into a laptop or tablet PC at the same time. Some providers appreciate online references, but for reluctant adopters, this is not a selling point.

7. Storing data off-site in more than one location is referred to as which of the following?

    A. Duplication
    B. Redundancy
    C. Virtual storage
    D. Archival storage

Storing data off-site in more than one location is referred to as redundancy. Redundant data storage ensures that if something happens to one data server, another one with the same data exists. Duplications, virtual storage, and archival storage are not terms for storing data in more than one location.

8. When removing computer equipment from service that once contained PHI, which of the following is accepted as a guarantee for preventing a privacy breach?

    A. Deleting all files
    B. Running a software scrub utility
    C. Disassembling and recycling the computer parts
    D. Reusing the equipment as long as it remains in the original facility

Deleting all files does not guarantee the removal of PHI. An EHR specialist has to delete the files and then run a software scrub utility to ensure PHI removal. Disassembling parts of the computer may include the hard drive, which may have PHI stored on it. Therefore, this is not an option without the EHR specialist first running a software scrub utility. A facility should not reuse the equipment without appropriately removing any PHI and applying the software scrub utility.

9. A provider's office that routinely submits reimbursement claims for allergy-related coughing as chronic asthma may be committing which of the following?

    A. Plagiarism
    B. Upcoding
    C. Medical malpractice
    D. Coding malpractice

Upcoding is the act of coding for a higher level diagnosis or service to receive higher reimbursement. It is illegal to upcode claims, either intentionally or accidently. Plagiarism is copying someone else's work and submitting it as your own. Medical malpractice refers to actions a provider takes. Poor coding practices are not defined as malpractice.

Terms and Definitions

Ad hoc reports – Reports created or programmed in response to an inquiry or issue that comes up; they are not normally scheduled reports

Compliance – Compliance as it relates to paper or electronic medical records refers to the completion of the record and the adherence to medical records and documentation requirements set forth by state and federal law, as well as accreditation and regulatory agencies

Database queries – Reports run on records stored in a database to find specific information; an ad hoc report is set up as a query

Diagnosis-related groups (DRGs) – Assigned to inpatients based on the principal diagnosis; determines the hospital's reimbursement; based on the prospective payment system

Garbage-in, garbage-out (GIGO) – Refers to the fact that poor documentation or data entry results in poor output from a computer or information system

Incomplete charts – Charts that are missing signatures, reports, or other required elements as outlined in either CMS Conditions for Participation for Medical Record Services or the Joint Commission accreditation guidelines for information management

Payers – Another word for insurance companies or the responsible party who will pay for the medical services patients receive; when patients do not have insurance, the payer listed on the bill is self-pay

Point-of-care (POC) charting – The ability of providers to document the care and treatment they render in real time, when they are with the patient; it is made much easier with the use of clinical templates, digital dictation, point-and-click menus, and other technology solutions

Record destruction policy – Facilities that maintain medical records of any form must have a record destruction policy in place; an attorney should guide the development of any policy on records and consider state and federal laws, along with any regulatory and accreditation requirements

Record retention – How long to retain medical records is a policy decision based on state and federal laws and regulatory and accreditation agency guidelines; an attorney should guide the development of any policy and consider facility needs that include patient characteristics, demographics, type of facility, and the availability of archived records and how that meets provider and patient needs

Redundant data storage – Storing data from your facility in more than one location so if one area is hit with a disaster event, the data is restored from a copy located elsewhere

Reimbursement – Payment for services rendered; refers to the end result of the revenue cycle

Revenue cycle – Five-step process that begins with providing services; after delivering services, providers document the care in the patient record, which drives the assignment of a code and establishes charges so a claim or bill can be prepared, submitted, and eventually, revenue received

Upcoding – Intentional or unintentional assignment of a higher level code than the documentation supports

Vendor – Company or organization that sold a product or service to a facility; in EHR technology issues, EHR specialists should keep communications open with the vendor so they can work jointly to quickly resolve issues around software updates, hardware or software problems, or new functionality

04 REGULATORY COMPLIANCE

Learning Objectives

After reading this chapter, you will be able to:

- *Adhere to professional standards of care as they pertain to medical records.*

- *Maintain confidentiality of protected health information (PHI) in compliance with HIPAA's Privacy Rule and your facility's policy.*

- *Maintain security of PHI in compliance with HIPAA's Security Rule and your facility's policy.*

- *Detect and reconcile threats to the security of electronic information.*

- *Audit compliance and report to the proper enforcement officer.*

- *Release PHI in accordance with HIPAA and your facility's policy.*

- *Participate in internal audits of medical records, such as consent forms and Release of Information (ROI) forms.*

- *Comply with patient safety standards regarding abbreviations in a health information system.*

- *Execute a plan for data recovery in the case of a catastrophic event.*

- *De-identify PHI when directed.*

Introduction

Everyone who works with medical records strives to provide accurate and consistent documentation to support the provision of quality health care and remain in compliance with legal and regulatory requirements, which are critical to the health care delivery system. State and federal law, CMS, and accreditation agencies specify standards of professional care in managing patient records. As an EHR specialist, you will play a key role in meeting these standards and maintaining high quality documentation practices for your facility.

Adhere to Professional Standards of Care as They Pertain to Medical Records

Handling a person's most private and personal information is a serious responsibility. Think about your own personal health history for just a minute and ask yourself how you might feel if others treated it carelessly or shared it indiscriminately whether unintentionally or maliciously.

The **American Health Information Management Association (AHIMA)** is one of the organizations most prominent in establishing a code of ethics for the handling of health information. Health care professionals who belong to this organization are bound by a code of ethics, which outlines professional standards anyone with access to personal health data can use as a guide.

With respect to the protection of the information within each record, an EHR specialist has the obligation to protect all patient health information in any format and to take any necessary precautions to prevent access to the information by unauthorized individuals. This caution applies to more than the patient's illness or injury. Best practices and professional standards require all information from the patient record be treated as highly sensitive, including personal information, financial information, any reference to genetic data, and outcome information, which includes when a patient dies, moves into a long-term care facility, or returns home. All of this information is private, and an EHR specialist and others working in the health care field should work to protect it from those who should not see it.

In addition to protecting privacy and confidentiality of patient records, another important professional standard of care involves properly handling the information to protect its integrity. The medical record, regardless of its format, is the legal record of a patient's care as provided by the professionals who document that care within the record. As such, you need to prevent any data loss or corruption of the medical record. As an EHR specialist, you will not document patient care in the record. However, you may at times come across entries in the record that are incorrect or incomplete. You must follow professional standards of care when addressing these findings and guide the clinical staff in these same standards.

You should never **delete** information or entries in a medical record, regardless of the reason. Documentation mistakes happen. They may include documenting the incorrect care, a wrong medication dose, or clinician advice that does not apply to that patient. In the paper record, the clinician should correct an error in the appropriate and legal way by drawing a single line through the incorrect record entry and writing the word ERROR above it. The original entry must still be readable but marked as erroneous. Then, the clinician writes the correct information in the record, noting that it is a correction to previous data and taking care to sign and date this entry. As a legal document of care, it is critical all information be available for review, either by medical professionals who need to understand everything that took place – right or wrong – or by legal professionals deciding on the validity of a malpractice claim against a provider, hospital, or other health care entity.

In both paper and electronic records, a clinician may need to enter new or additional information to documentation for a number of reasons. If the clinician adds information that was left out of the original entry, this is an **addendum**. If the clinician needs to add clarification or details missing from the initial documentation, she would make an **amendment** to the record. Amendments add additional information that may serve to clarify the original notes but should not change the general information in the record. Other add-on documentation includes **corrections** and **late entries**. Corrections may include changing the report from describing the patient as a 10-year-old male to a 10-year-old female, due to a transcription mistake, while late entries include anything a clinician documents after the fact. An example of a late entry would be if a nurse performs a dressing change on a patient at the end of his shift but forgets to chart this task. In the morning when he returns to work, he may add the late entry about the dressing change to the patient record. Late entries are not ideal, and the clinical staff should avoid them as often as possible.

As you become familiar with the software in your facility, you will learn how clinicians handle updates, errors, and additional information in the electronic record. As an EHR specialist, you can help them understand that one of the risks to corrections or updates in an EHR is that, unlike a paper entry where the word ERROR is plainly seen in the documentation, an addendum or other update note in and EHR may appear just like other documentation in the text of the record. Be sure to familiarize yourself with the policy in your facility so you can properly audit patient records for compliance.

In rare cases, you may encounter patients who wish to remove an entry or information from their record. While the information in the record technically belongs to the patient, the record itself is a business document that belongs to the facility, and you should never remove information from it. If a patient is adamant that an entry in his record is an error, take his name and contact information and tell him you will let the clinician know. In most cases, you will want to notify the clinician who wrote the entry in question. If this is not possible, ask another clinician in your facility how best to handle the situation. In no circumstance should you engage with the patient in an argumentative way. Thank the patient for bringing it to your attention; tell him you cannot remove anything from a record; and assure him you will alert the clinician of his concerns and get back to him. In some facilities there may be a policy in place that allows patients, or their legal representatives, to add their own entry to the medical record. This would not replace the clinician documentation but would represent the patient's perspective on the matter on the record.

In the outpatient and inpatient setting, health care professionals handle sensitive, highly personal, and private information that is critically important to quality patient care. Take this responsibility seriously as an important step in your personal and professional development.

Maintain Confidentiality of PHI in Compliance with HIPAA Privacy Rule and Facility Policy

In 1996, HIPAA became law. Although this legislation is broader than simply health information privacy, the term "HIPAA" is now synonymous with privacy and security of health information.

At the time, the U.S. Congress had concerns about the emerging electronic environment in which many businesses were actively participating. The concerns about health information in this electronic environment became the foundation for the eventual HIPAA legislation, which includes rules for maintaining the privacy of patient health information, as well as protecting its security when transmitting or storing the information electronically. An important distinction between the HIPAA Privacy Rule and the HIPAA Security Rule is that the Privacy Rule defines privacy practices for and pertaining to all PHI in any format – spoken, written, or electronic – whereas the Security Rule is specific to health information that is in an electronic format.

When you fax a paper record to an authorized user, the information transforms from a static, paper-based format to an electronic format. Faxing patient information falls under the protection of the HIPAA Security Rule. You may want to discuss how to encrypt fax information with your Information Technology department. It is important to become familiar with your state's privacy and security laws regarding PHI because they may be more stringent than the federal HIPAA laws. There may also be more stringent laws when dealing with drug and alcohol, mental illness, and HIV/AIDs patient information. In all cases, follow the more "strict" law.

When considering the privacy of health information, it is important to think about more than locking doors or computer logins as the way to protect patient information. Consider conversations you may have with colleagues or others in the course of a day. Are you talking about a patient or information you saw in a patient record? Not only is it possible for others to overhear your discussion, but if you are not working directly with the patient record at that time, you have no need to share the information with a colleague, especially outside of the department or work space.

Use this simple formula for making decisions on what to share in the workplace as it relates to patient information: Is sharing this information necessary for the performance of your job duties? If the answer is no, then ask if sharing the information is necessary for someone else in the facility to accomplish his or her job duties? If the answer to this is also no, then you should keep the information to yourself. Avoid the habit of finding great interest in the details of patients' information and look at the data as a tool you work with to perform your job. Lastly, if temptation to share something particularly interesting overtakes you, stop and pretend that the details are about you or someone you care about. Then imagine someone you do not like discussing those details with great interest.

Maintain Security of PHI in Compliance with HIPAA Security Rule and Facility Policy

Electronic health records reside behind firewalls and should require a unique login and password, along with the appropriate rights to access them. Sometimes this layer of electronic protection causes people to forget the basics of security, which includes locking doors to rooms and departments with computers or servers in them. Another area of concern involves mobile devices, such as laptops, mobile phones, and tablets, that contain PHI. Keep these devices in a secure location to prevent them from being tampered with or stolen.

In facilities that remain largely paper-based, privacy and security may seem fairly simple. Locking doors is a primary and important security precaution. It is also important to have strict policies and procedures in place for accessing records. On one hand, paper records seem simpler to manage than electronic records because generally, a medical records department has one main area to secure for medical charts and records. On the other hand, as charts leave to go out into patient care units and outpatient clinics, the controls pertaining to the medical records or HIM department are harder to enforce.

Electronic health records also present privacy challenges. Employees working with PHI on a computer must remember never to walk away while their computer is logged into the system. Most computers enable you to set up an auto-lock if no activity occurs for a set period of time. For inpatient environments, the IT department will likely have a policy about logins and may have already set up the auto-lock feature. For outpatient settings, you may need to suggest this as an improvement to security for patient information.

The first rule to maintaining this electronic security is to never share your **password** with anyone. Do not write it down and put it in a convenient place. Intruders know where to look for such things. They will check for notes under keyboards, desks, and on bulletin boards behind the monitor screen. Memorize your password and do not write it down. Many facilities have a password rotation requirement. These range from rotating your password every 90 days to twice a year or annually. Most rotations do not allow users to activate a password that was in use three changes ago. It's imperative that passwords are complex and hard to guess. Avoid using simple passwords such as "1234," "abcd," or "password." The more varied the mix of letters, numbers, and special characters, the harder your password is to crack. Passwords are generally eight characters long, but some security experts recommend even longer ones. Examples of strong passwords might include "5un5h!n3" or "@pp134me." You may think these are hard to remember. However, if you think of "'5un5h!n3' as a play on the word "sunshine," or "@pp134me" as "apple for me," you can make an appropriately strong password easy to remember.

As an EHR specialist, you can model appropriate computer security behavior and provide expert guidance to others in your workplace to make patient information as safe as possible.

Detect Threats to the Security of Electronic Information

As you already know, one of the most important and often overlooked aspects of information security is simply locking rooms that contain computers and other technology. In an ideal world, doors would never be left open, but mistakes happen. If you see someone you do not know hanging around or coming out of a computer room or patient file area that is normally locked, ask her if she needs assistance. If she seems nervous or agitated or is calm but cannot show you a facility ID, the information systems may be at risk, which means patient information is at risk. Contact your facility's privacy officer. If you are working in a small provider's office or clinic without a designated privacy officer, let the office manager or someone else in charge know about the incident. Depending on the setup of your system, you may want to call the electronic medical record (EMR) host or the company hosting your servers. The best time to locate this information is before an incident. Make sure you are familiar with the specific rules and regulations in your facility so you can respond in an appropriate manner in case of a potential privacy or security breach.

Other threats to the security of patient electronic information may be less obvious and require more sophisticated tools. **Audit trails** are one such tool. An audit trail is a record of system activity. It provides detailed reporting on user access and activity into systems, applications, and processes and is an important part of any health care facility's information security plan.

In most hospitals, the system of audit trails is set up and managed by the IT department in consultation with the privacy officer. In smaller facilities, clinics, or providers' offices, this may be an internal task or one the remote server host or EMR vendor manages and then sends the reports to your facility. As an EHR specialist, you may find your role includes reviewing these reports on a daily or weekly basis.

You know about RBACs from your reading earlier in the study guide. You may recall that RBACs assign specific access rights to each person in the facility who has a login ID and a password. However, RBACs are not fool-proof. Careful review of the audit trail reports can reveal information you or others need to identify inappropriate access.

Work with your IT department, your EMR software vendor, or other experts to put the best security practices in place. Also work with your team to implement the industry standards for password rotation, and teach colleagues about the basics of protecting access to electronic patient information. Most importantly, remember that privacy and security are everyone's job when working with PHI.

Reconcile Threats to the Security of Electronic Information

Taking quick action when a weakness in security or a breach occurs is critical. When you identify a potential problem area, take steps to identify if it is an existing problem or one that is newly emerging as a threat to the security of your patients' health information.

In a hospital or inpatient setting, report any threats to the security of electronic information or systems to the IT department. These professionals manage the networks, passwords, and information systems and are in the best position to take action when a potential problem comes to light.

In smaller clinics or provider's office settings, the role of an EHR specialist may require more specific steps before handing the issue off to the IT professionals. If, for example, your facility uses a single login and password for everyone to access the system, you can suggest a new policy of individual, unique user logins and passwords, along with a password rotation schedule. Work with your colleagues to make the transition smooth. Be sure to explain why this is important and how it helps to protect your patients' information. You may also find that some of your colleagues walk away from their computers without logging off, leaving open access to the system and records. Again, your knowledge and guidance in these matters can help change behaviors that put everyone at risk.

Learning the system in your workplace and the use patterns of colleagues and other authorized users can help you develop best practices for securing the information in your facility and protecting your patients' privacy.

Audit Compliance and Report to Proper Enforcement Officer

Reporting compliance violations will be specific to each facility. They may involve the HIM department in one hospital and the IT department in another. In larger facilities, a **Compliance Officer** handles issues relating to information security compliance and will often lead a compliance committee that has representatives from across the facility, such as nursing, HIM, laboratory, emergency, and other departments. Some of the tasks charged to the Compliance Officer and the committee include: performing periodic risk assessments and developing appropriate response plans to identified risks, internal monitoring and auditing, such as receiving and reviewing audit trail reports, responding to any identified breach of information systems security, developing a plan for corrective action, and reporting all findings to the government as required by law. While compliance and privacy duties often combine into a single position, such Privacy Compliance Officer in hospitals and health care systems, smaller facilities usually identify someone as the **Privacy Official**, who, in addition to regular job duties, has privacy duties and must be familiar with the HIPAA and HITECH provisions that govern the management of patients' PHI.

After any discovery of a breach of PHI, the covered entity, such as providers, hospitals, or clinics, must notify individuals whose information is at risk, as well as the Secretary of the Department of Health and Human Services (HHS), and, in some cases, the media. The Office of Civil Rights, a division of HHS, enforces HIPAA regulations.

As an EHR specialist, you may participate in a Compliance Committee or be the point person in your department who relays compliance issues to the committee. In smaller facilities, you may work with the office manager or clinic business manager who serves as the Privacy Official to address privacy and compliance issues. Regardless of the environment, it is important to familiarize yourself with the HITECH Act breach notification rules and stay informed about updates, additions, and new processes pertaining to the collection, storage, management, and release of PHI.

Release PHI in Accordance with HIPAA and Facility Policy

One of the most common activities the privacy rule governs involves the release of information. The HIPAA Privacy Rule includes clear guidelines for the release of health information with the goal of limiting the disclosure of PHI as much as possible. The Privacy Rule outlines only two cases where release of information is required: when a patient or his legal representative requests access to his information and in response to a HHS investigation.

Other circumstances permit the release of PHI without specific authorization and include the following: when a patient requests a copy of her information; to support treatment, payment, or operational health care activities; and in compliance with certain public health and legal guidelines, such as in reporting sexually transmitted disease or suspected cases of abuse and neglect.

For a release of information that requires the patient's authorization, be sure you document all of the items necessary to make it legal. This includes the patient's full name, which information to release, such as the entire record or all records from a specific episode or time period, the person or entity receiving the record, and an expiration date for the authorization.

In facilities or circumstances where the patient record or information is sensitive in nature, such as in the case of psychiatric, HIV/AIDS, or substance abuse records, check state law to ensure you are in compliance with any special requirements for releasing this information.

It is also helpful to remember the **minimum necessary standard**, which as part of the HIPAA Privacy Rule mandates covered entities release only information that pertains to the request. Consider a hypothetical female patient who has been in the hospital twice for gynecological health issues. She then breaks her leg in three places and is in the hospital for more than a month. After discharge, she requests documentation regarding why she can no longer work in a job where she stands all day. In this case, the minimum necessary standard would indicate the facility release only the records relating to her leg injury for this request.

Patients rely on informed health care professionals to guide them according to applicable laws and what is in their best interest. Knowing the laws and how they apply to the tasks in your facility safeguards patients' private health data and protects you, your colleagues, and facility from violating federal and state privacy laws.

Participate in Internal Audits of Medical Records

Regular audits are the best way to know your facility is in compliance with the many regulatory and legal requirements for medical records and patient information. As you know, CMS and the Joint Commission require that certain reports appear in the medical record within a specified time frame. EHR technology and the nature of discrete or structured data in the electronic record make quick work of querying for missing history and physical reports, unsigned orders, and outstanding discharge summaries. In hospitals and larger facilities, these reports are likely run on a regular schedule. **Consent forms** are also an important part of the medical record and both the physician and the patient must sign the form, along with a witness, before providers render any medical treatment. A provider that treats a patient without consent may be liable for criminal charges of **battery** if the patient or her family disagree with the treatment or are unhappy with the outcome.

Advance directives allow patients to make decisions about their current or future health care. They also facilitate the assignment of decision-making authority to another person who can then make health care decisions if the patient can no longer do so. Advance directives may appear in the record as a living will, a do-not-resuscitate (DNR) order, right-to-die documentation, or durable powers of attorney. The **Patient Self-Determination Act (PSDA)** mandates that patients receive information on their rights to determine their course of care when admitting them to a hospital or other health care facility, which excludes provider's office encounters. While it is against the law to require a patient to have advance directives, hospitals must inform patients of their rights to advance directives. As an EHR specialist, you may verify the hospital's compliance by checking for documentation of discussions about advance directives in the nurse's progress notes or for the presence of advance directives in the record. In EHR systems, there may be a check-box option the clinician may select when a patient receives advance directives information. For hospitals, Stage 1 Meaningful Use includes the measure of how many patients, age 65 and older, have advance directives documented in their medical record. This documentation could include a living will, durable powers of attorney, or simply the acknowledgement the patient is aware of his rights and his ability to document advance directives upon admission.

Consents for treatment in the outpatient setting are similar to those in hospitals and other care settings and are equally important. The same standards for release of information apply to the outpatient office, and the process is the same as for hospitals and other facilities. It is also important to provide each patient with a Notice of Privacy Practices for Protected Health information. Facilities may distribute this in print or electronic format. At the time, ask patients to sign a form, acknowledging their receipt of the privacy notice. Many practices are using electronic signature pads to capture this documentation after patients read the privacy notification on a computer. This eliminates the need to print reams of paper that end up in the trash.

Lastly, checking for a patients' signature on file can ensure your facility can provide payment directly to your provider. Providers may have patients fill out an authorization to bill for services and sign it for the provider to keep on file. Then, when submitting claims for reimbursement, the provider can indicate "Signature on File" on the forms. This informs the third-party payer or insurance company that the patient authorizes the provider to receive insurance payments directly. Signature on File generally remains in place for multiple claims. Check with your facility for the timetable for updating patient signatures. Signature on File saves time and paperwork with each office visit and ensures payers will not hold up reimbursement waiting for a new signature with each claim.

Comply with Patient Safety Standards Regarding Abbreviations

The Joint Commission's **National Patient Safety Goals** became public only one year after the release of the dangerous abbreviations and "Do Not Use" list, which is specific to abbreviations in the paper-based medical record. The list of forbidden abbreviations includes many that are easily mistaken for other abbreviations with dangerous outcomes. Some examples include U for unit, IU for international units, and the traditional Latin abbreviations for daily (Q.D. or q.d.) and every other day (Q.O.D. and q.o.d.). Poor handwriting can confuse these notations, making them impossible to decipher and dangerous to patients. $MgSO_4$ and MSO_4 are so close but drastically different in their use. $MgSO_4$ is the chemical formula for magnesium sulfate, while MSO_4 indicates morphine sulfate. Administering morphine instead of magnesium has the potential to cause harm.

Initially the Do Not Use list was not required in computerized patient records. Currently, these prohibitions apply to orders and medication-related documentation that is handwritten or on pre-printed forms. It also applies to free-text computer entries. Some facilities keep a list of approved abbreviations. This can be quite long and leaves them open to scrutiny by accreditation and licensing agencies. If an approved list exists, all abbreviations in use by any clinician must appear there, whereas maintaining only a **Do Not Use** list of abbreviations is much more manageable. Electronic health records and computer-assisted documentation is changing the conversation about abbreviations and other handwriting-related issues. As an EHR specialist, you may find it necessary to address the issue, so it is best to stay up to date on this important issue.

Execute a Plan for Data Recovery in the Case of a Catastrophic Event

Catastrophic events are never pleasant, but careful planning can help everyone get back in business as soon as possible. This is true for individuals, families, and the professionals who manage volumes of detailed health information.

You do not need to search far to find a news story about a hurricane, tornado, flood, or fire somewhere in the country. These weather events and other catastrophic events present major challenges for health records and, without proper planning, can wreak havoc long after the disaster event is finished.

In Chapter 1, you read about backing up EHR data. This is necessary whether or not you anticipate a catastrophic event, but, in the case of a disaster, it is helpful to have a sturdy plan for data recovery and to practice it on a regular basis.

You know how important patient records are for providing continuity of care and acting as a legal record for your facility. Any backup and storage options must address the complex information systems, as well as legal and ethical requirements for protecting patient health information.

One common theme from people who have come through a disaster event with patient records intact is the staunch support for putting all records online. Paper records can disintegrate in a flood, disappear in a tornado, or burn in a fire. Having the ability to purchase new laptops and log in to your off-site remote data storage location or access your EMR data through the web allows a facility to be back in business in as little as a few days, even after a major catastrophe.

Some of the recommended practices for data backup and recovery in a disaster include:

- **Redundancy**: Have more than one, and possibly several, copies of your data. This is often done by mirroring servers in multiple locations. Mirroring means the data is the same on each server.

- Storing off-site data geographically away from your place of business to keep the likelihood of the same disaster event wiping out your data and your backup data minimal.

- Stay up to date on data storage options and recovery best practices. In most cases, these tasks will be assigned to the IT professionals who are responsible for managing the information system.

- Practice restoring your data at least once a year. Schedule practices on a weekend and involve your EMR vendor or IT experts. Your first attempt at a data restore should not happen after a disaster.

- Consult with your EMR vendor or IT consultants on a regular basis. This field changes rapidly, and your data is too important to manage with old technology.

Patients trust health care professionals to put their best interests first. Start by planning for data recovery in any scenario and safeguarding the documentation providers rely on to provide the best patient care.

De-identify PHI when Directed

Health records contain valuable information, not only for patients but for researchers, public health organizations, and registries. The challenge in releasing the information from health records focuses on the protection of patient identity, while meeting the needs of secondary data users. As an EHR specialist, you may be asked to pull data from the EHR databases to submit to a disease registry, such as a diabetes registry or immunization registry, or to gather information for researchers or other public health requests.

To **de-identify** PHI according to the HIPAA Privacy Rule, remove the following elements from the record or data:

- All names

- All geographic subdivisions smaller than a state

- All dates (except year) directly applicable to an individual

- Telephone numbers

- Fax numbers

- Email addresses

- Social Security numbers

- Medical record numbers

- Health plan beneficiary numbers

- Account numbers

- Certificate/license numbers

- Vehicle identifiers and serial numbers, including license plate numbers

- Device identifiers and serial numbers

- Web URLs

- IP addresses

- Biometric identifiers, including fingerprints and voiceprints

- Full-face photographs or images

- Any other unique identifying numbers, characteristics, or codes, unless otherwise permitted

De-identified health information does not need patient authorization for release, although, as a matter of practice, some facilities ask all patients to sign releases indicating their information is available for use by researchers. This blanket authorization allows researchers quicker access to patient information that potentially contains PHI, which in some circumstances can be important, such as epidemiologists evaluating a viral outbreak by zip code.

De-identified health information plays an important role in supporting research and education. As an EHR specialist, learning how to identify when patient data is properly de-identified and then releasing it to the appropriate group or individual contributes to the improvements in health care, communities, and society overall.

Summary

Learning the intricate rules and regulations for proper management of patient information is an important role for an EHR specialist. With technological advancements providing more open opportunities to information and legal and regulatory requirements seeking to narrow access, the competing and often conflicting demands on health care data are complex and ever-changing.

In your role, it is important to stay up to date with regulatory mandates, such as those from CMS and the Joint Commission. It is also a good idea to keep regular communication channels open with IT professionals whose knowledge on best practices in data storage, protection, and recovery are vital to those managing health records.

You must also recognize threats to patient privacy and the security of information in your care. Be ready to act to protect your patients by notifying the appropriate official, making changes that will prevent unauthorized access, such as locking doors and keeping your password private, and helping your colleagues and others employ the safest information management practices.

Drill Questions

1. An EHR specialist is coaching a new physician's assistant on documentation standards for the patient record. Which of the following actions by the assistant requires further teaching?

    A. Charting a late entry
    B. Appending a progress note
    C. Deleting incorrect data from a record
    D. Correcting inaccurate data in a record

2. A provider emails patient information to a surgeon's office. Which of the following pertains specifically to emailed information?

    A. HIPAA Security Rule
    B. Patient Self Determination Act (PSDA)
    C. HIPAA Privacy Rule
    D. National Patient Safety Goals

3. An EHR specialist is creating a password. Which of the following describes a password that is hard to crack by potential system intruders?

    A. His mother's maiden name
    B. A combination of letters, numbers, and special characters
    C. His Social Security number
    D. A combination of upper and lower case letters

4. A nurse on the Medical-Surgical unit believes someone used her login and password on a day she was not at work. An EHR specialist should perform which of the following actions to investigate this issue?

    A. Check the audit trail.
    B. Question other employees who worked that day.
    C. Run a network scan.
    D. Submit a report to the compliance committee.

5. The "Do Not Use" list serves to prevent the use of which of the following?

    A. Words that are not appropriate in the patient record
    B. Software tools that are not HIPAA Security Rule compliant
    C. Medications that are no longer on the market for patient use
    D. Abbreviations that have the potential to be confusing

6. An EHR specialist is delivering an audit trail report to a nursing supervisor on the 8th floor. While waiting at the elevator to return to the HIM department, she notices a woman with a small child, standing at a COW and typing into the keyboard. Just as the EHR specialist was about to confront her, the woman grabs her child's hand and heads in the other direction. Which of the following is an appropriate action for the EHR specialist to take?

   A. Let her supervisor know when she returns to the department.
   B. Return to the nursing station to see if the woman works there.
   C. Contact the hospital's Privacy Official.
   D. Call a law enforcement authority.

7. Which of the following is recommended to ensure data recovery after a disaster?

   A. Maintain duplicate servers to provide data redundancy.
   B. Back up to tapes that are locked in the safe on site.
   C. Back up to tapes that are taken home by the office manager each night.
   D. Keep a paper copy of each patient's record as a backup.

8. An older adult comes into the hospital as a patient and tells the admitting provider he wants his son to make all of his decisions. Which of the following should the provider give the family regarding this request?

   A. Consent forms for treatment
   B. Signature on File form
   C. Minimum necessary standard form
   D. Advance directives form

9. A 35-year-old man has a history of hospital admissions for kidney stones. He is admitted through the emergency department following a motor vehicle crash. Several months later, an attorney's office calls the HIM department and requests a copy of the patient's medical record because the patient is pressing charges against the other driver in the crash. The patient has signed a release of information authorization for his treatment relating to the accident. Which of the following is important for the EHR specialist to remember when processing this record request?

   A. Patient Self Determination Act (PSDA)
   B. Checking for advance directives
   C. Minimum necessary standard
   D. De-identifying patient information

10. A patient is having surgery on her hip. Which of the following must be in the record before the surgery begins?

    A. Advance directives
    B. Consent form
    C. Powers of attorney documentation
    D. Record addendum

Drill Answers

1. An EHR specialist is coaching a new physician's assistant on documentation standards for the patient record. Which of the following actions by the assistant requires further teaching?

   A. Charting a late entry
   B. Appending a progress note
   C. Deleting incorrect data from a record
   D. Correcting inaccurate data in a record

   It is not appropriate to delete information from a legal document, such as a health record. Charting a late entry is not ideal, but late entries are acceptable. Appending progress notes is acceptable. Correcting erroneous data is acceptable as long as the original entries remain in the record.

2. A provider emails patient information to a surgeon's office. Which of the following pertains specifically to emailed information?

   A. HIPAA Security Rule
   B. Patient Self Determination Act (PSDA)
   C. HIPAA Privacy Rule
   D. National Patient Safety Goals

   The HIPAA Security Rule addresses the transmission, storage, and capture of PHI through electronic means. The PSDA has nothing to do with sending PHI via email. The HIPAA Privacy Rule addresses the privacy protections for all patient information, but it does not specifically address transfer of PHI. The National Patient Safety Goals do not address sending PHI via email.

3. An EHR specialist is creating a password. Which of the following describes a password that is hard to crack by potential system intruders?

   A. His mother's maiden name
   B. A combination of letters, numbers, and special characters
   C. His Social Security number
   D. A combination of upper and lower case letters

   A combination of letters, numbers, and special characters describes a password that is hard to crack by potential system intruders. The more complex the password, the harder it is to crack or guess. Simple names that can be accessed easily, such as the EHR specialist's mother's maiden name, are not good passwords. It is not appropriate for the EHR specialist to use his Social Security number as his password. While a combination of upper and lower case letters is better than a simple password, such as "1234" or "abcd," a password that includes letters, numbers, and special characters is best.

4. A nurse on the Medical-Surgical unit believes someone used her login and password on a day she was not at work. An EHR specialist should perform which of the following actions to investigate this issue?

> **A. Check the audit trail.**
> B. Question other employees who worked that day.
> C. Run a network scan.
> D. Submit a report to the compliance committee.

> **The audit trail will show if the nurse was logged in that day and from which computers. It will also show any data areas or applications that were in use during the login. Questioning other employees who worked that day and running a network scan are not efficient or appropriate actions to investigate this issue. While a report to the compliance committee may come later, it is not how the EHR specialist should investigate whether there was a breach or not.**

5. The "Do Not Use" list serves to prevent the use of which of the following?

> A. Words that are not appropriate in the patient record
> B. Software tools that are not HIPAA Security Rule compliant
> C. Medications that are no longer on the market for patient use
> **D. Abbreviations that have the potential to be confusing**

> **The "Do Not Use" list notes confusing and potentially dangerous abbreviations the clinical staff should avoid when documenting patient care.**

6. An EHR specialist is delivering an audit trail report to a nursing supervisor on the 8th floor. While waiting at the elevator to return to the HIM department, she notices a woman with a small child, standing at a COW and typing into the keyboard. Just as the EHR specialist was about to confront her, the woman grabs her child's hand and heads in the other direction. Which of the following is an appropriate action for the EHR specialist to take?

> A. Let her supervisor know when she returns to the department.
> B. Return to the nursing station to see if the woman works there.
> **C. Contact the hospital's Privacy Official.**
> D. Call a law enforcement authority.

> **The EHR specialist should contact the hospital's Privacy Official immediately.**

7. Which of the following is recommended to ensure data recovery after a disaster?

    A. Maintain duplicate servers to provide data redundancy.
    B. Back up to tapes that are locked in the safe on site.
    C. Back up to tapes that are taken home by the office manager each night.
    D. Keep a paper copy of each patient's record as a backup.

Maintaining duplicate servers to provide data redundancy is the best practice to ensure data recovery after a disaster. If the facility backs up tapes and keeps them locked in an on-site safe these tapes would be destroyed. Backing up tapes and having the office manager take them home each night is not the best practice to ensure data recovery after a disaster. Keeping a paper copy of each patient's record as a backup is not practical and defeats the purpose of electronic records.

8. An older adult comes into the hospital as a patient and tells the admitting provider he wants his son to make all of his decisions. Which of the following should the provider give the family regarding this request?

    A. Consent forms for treatment
    B. Signature on File form
    C. Minimum necessary standard form
    D. Advance directives form

The option of designating powers of attorney is part of advance directives. Consent forms agree to the proposed treatment or care. Signature on File forms help providers receive payment quicker. The minimum necessary standard relates to the release of patient information.

9. A 35-year-old man has a history of hospital admissions for kidney stones. He is admitted through the emergency department following a motor vehicle crash. Several months later, an attorney's office calls the HIM department and requests a copy of the patient's medical record because the patient is pressing charges against the other driver in the crash. The patient has signed a release of information authorization for his treatment relating to the accident. Which of the following is important for the EHR specialist to remember when processing this record request?

    A. Patient Self Determination Act (PSDA)
    B. Checking for advance directives
    C. Minimum necessary standard
    D. De-identifying patient information

The minimum necessary standard of the HIPAA Privacy Rule dictates only information necessary to fulfill the intent of the request be sent. The PSDA has nothing to do with the release of records. Advance directives have nothing to do with the release of records. The EHR specialist would not de-identify patient information in this kind of record.

10. A patient is having surgery on her hip. Which of the following must be in the record before the surgery begins?

    A. Advance directives
    B. Consent form
    C. Powers of attorney documentation
    D. Record addendum

Performing any treatment on a patient without consent is battery and against the law. Advance directives, powers of attorney documentation, and a record addendum are not required before a surgery.

Terms and Definitions

Addendum – Additional documentation added to a health record that represents new data not included in the original documentation

Advance directives – Documents that give patients the right to make decisions about their care and designate others to make decisions if they are incapacitated

Amendment – An addition to patient record documentation meant to clarify or further explain existing record information

American Health Information Management Association (AHIMA) – The national organization for medical records professionals

Audit trails – A computer software program that tracks users by login and documents where in an information system users go and which applications they access

Battery – A legal term; harmful or offensive touching of another

Compliance Officer – A health care administrator charged with overseeing all compliance activities in the facility; often also serves as the privacy officer

Consent forms – Forms patients sign to give permission for treatment

Corrections – Entries in a patient health record that correct or change original data

De-identify – The stripping of any identifying pieces of data from health records so they can be used in research, education, or other public health activities

Delete – Removing data or information from the health record; this is not permitted

Late entries – Documentation added to the patient record after the care was provided

Minimum necessary standard – The HIPAA standard that requires covered entities to release only the minimum amount of patient health data to meet the need of the request

National Patient Safety Goals – Implemented by the Joint Commission in 2002, these goals focus on practices to safeguard patients in the health care delivery system; one example is the universal protocol, which requires a time out before any surgical procedure to verify right patient, right side, right procedure, etc.

Password – A unique set of characters, letters, and numbers that is kept private and allows users with an appropriate login ID to access an information system

Patient Self-Determination Act (PSDA) – The legislation that gives patients the right to make decisions about their care and outcomes, including being left alone to die and not resuscitated if that is not their desire

Privacy Official – HIPAA-required individual who is the point person for any privacy concerns or complaints; leads the facility in communicating privacy practices and reviewing existing practices for compliance with privacy requirements

Redundancy – Duplication; generally refers to data

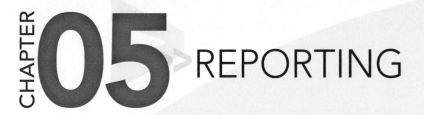

05 REPORTING

Learning Objectives

After reading this chapter, you will be able to:

- *Generate statistical reports for clinical quality improvement (QI) measures.*

- *Compile medical care and census data for continuity of care records.*

- *Generate statistical reports for financial QI measures.*

- *Generate aging reports by guarantor or carrier.*

- *Generate financial analysis reports by provider, diagnosis, or procedure.*

Introduction

Reporting health data and information is a major task for EHR specialists. You should understand the various data that most facilities collect, identify why it is collected, and recognize how the data reports help support the facilities providing quality patient care.

First, learn all the data locations and how to extract the data using database queries or software that is specific to your facility's information system. Learning why each data set is important and how it contributes to the advancement of quality in the health care delivery system allows you to spot patterns, trends, and anomalies, which is data that is out of place.

As regulatory and legal requirements expand, it's creating additional pressures on the health care delivery system. Your contributions to this extraction and management of data benefit your facility, the clinical staff – and ultimately – patients.

Generate Statistical Reports for Clinical Quality Improvement (QI) Measures

Quality is an important characteristic in any service a patient receives. At the end of the 20th century, the **Institute of Medicine (IOM)** reported as many as 98,000 patients were dying each year because of medical errors alone. The implementation of EHR software provided one solution to this problem. The Joint Commission and CMS also added clinical quality outcome measures to existing requirements. You play an important role in supporting quality initiatives by running and preparing these reports for use by the quality improvement team.

CMS and the Joint Commission require hospitals to collect and report data on specific diseases, procedures, or other outcomes to maintain their accredited status. The items under review represent patient categories that are known to be high-volume or high-risk. High-volume means a significant number of patients are presenting to hospitals and other health care facilities in these categories. Therefore, a significant amount of money goes into treating these patients. In the high-risk category, the diseases or procedures may not be large in number, but they represent a significant risk for each patient, as well as generating considerate health care expenses. The list of high-risk category diseases and procedures is evaluated over time and is not static. The **National Hospital Inpatient Quality Measures** includes a review of patients whose admission was due to diseases that include acute myocardial infarction (AMI), or heart attack, heart failure, pneumonia, or stroke. Asthma care in children is also a measure, as is data on the cause of death, or mortality measures, and readmission rates, or patients who return to the hospital within 30 days or less after discharge. For example, when patients present to a hospital with a principal diagnosis of acute myocardial infarction, the hospital collects data retrospectively, meaning they abstract the medical record after patient discharge. The hospital seeks out the following data:

- Did the patient receive aspirin at arrival?

- Did the patient receive an aspirin prescription or instructions to take aspirin at discharge?

- Did the patient receive an angiotensin-converting enzyme inhibitor or angiotensin receptor blockers if a left ventricular systolic dysfunction was present?

- Did the patient receive a prescription for a beta-blocker at discharge?

- What was the median time to fibrinolysis or how long did it take to administer across all AMI patients?

- Did the patient receive fibrinolytic therapy within 30 min of hospital arrival or how many AMI patients received the fibrinolytic therapy received within 30 min?

- What was the median time to primary percutaneous coronary intervention (PCI) for all AMI patients?

- By patient, how long did it take for the delivery of primary PCI?

- Did the patient receive a prescription for a statin, an anti-cholesterol medication, at discharge?

Review the list of data collection categories and the number of items to collect for each one. You will quickly see how you can help with collecting and reporting these important measures that identify the quality of care patients receive within your facility.

In many facilities, data on these indicators can appear in a graph using spreadsheet software. A common graph displays the hospital's performance on a quality measure in comparison with **benchmarks**, or target rates. The example below highlights the percentage of patients who were given aspirin at arrival.

You can see on this graph the line with the diamonds indicates the percentage of patients at this facility who received aspirin at arrival, as it compares to an internal benchmark the hospital set for itself, which is indicated by the line with the triangles, and as it compares to an external goal, which is indicated by the line with the squares. When evaluating

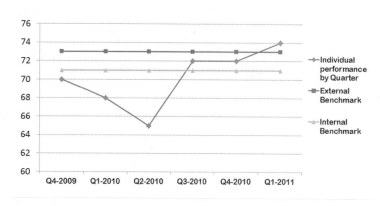

Benchmark example

quality of care, this type of data is critical to identifying what, how, and when the facility is meeting the expected patient care quality goals. Be sure to apply your knowledge of data queries and the location of various data items in the EHR to support your facility's path to quality care.

You might notice that the outpatient setting includes fewer formal reports. Even so, extracting data from the patient records remains important. With the CMS Meaningful Use program continuing through at least 2014, many provider offices and other smaller facility settings look to document their meaningful use of EHR technology, including clinical quality measures, such as documenting tobacco use, percentage of patients age 50 and older who receive a flu shot, and childhood immunization status.

Knowing the format and location of the data in the EMR your facility uses is a critical skill you should possess. Regardless of the environment you work in, make it an early priority to learn which quality measures the clinicians' need to evaluate and document and where the data resides in the electronic record. In doing this, you will not only support the meaningful use of EHR technology, but you will contribute to a higher quality experience for your facility's patients.

Compile Medical Care and Census Data for Continuity of Care Records

Hospitals often get a data-rich, but information-poor reputation. This refers to the volumes of data they collect, store, and churn through on a daily, weekly, monthly, quarterly, and yearly basis. This criticism is somewhat less relevant since the implementation of EHR technology, which makes it easier to pull data from thousands – even millions – of records in a short period of time.

Statistical and census data is historically the domain of the HIM department in hospitals. Common reports for inpatient settings include daily census, the number of patients in active hospital inpatient beds for a single 24-hr period; **total inpatient service days**, the number of inpatients receiving care each day totaled for the number of days in the report; **occupancy rate**, the percentage of active patient beds that have a patient assigned to them; and average length of stay, which is represented in days for inpatients; as well as more clinical data, including **mortality rates**, meaning death rates, **autopsy rates**, and **morbidity** rates, meaning disease rates.

Data that populates these and other reports serve a variety of purposes. The bed occupancy shows how many patients occupy beds in the facility. If there are too many empty beds, that indicates a low occupancy rate. If most beds are full, that indicates a high occupancy rate. **Daily census** reports are specific to each **patient care unit (PCU)** and show where patients are plentiful and where there are open beds. This data is useful not only for decisions on whether to close units or build an addition, but it can also assist in human resources planning for the addition or reduction of clinical staff. Facilities must report a number of the data items to the state, including death rates and birth rates, which in turn submits data known as vital statistics to a national data warehouse, such as the National Committee on Vital and Health Statistics (NCVHS). The NCVHS advises the **Department of Health and Human Services**, the **Centers for Disease Control and Prevention (CDC)**, and the **National Center for Health Statistics (NCHS)**.

Reporting is similar in the outpatient and inpatient environments. However, reporting is sometimes more difficult in the outpatient environment because of the variety of practice patterns among providers. The **National Ambulatory Medical Care Survey (NAMCS)** collects data regarding which outpatient services occur in provider offices and clinics that provide direct patient care. Your role in gathering and reporting this data is critical to meeting national reporting requirements, as well as documenting the care the clinical staff provides. This data reports on physician characteristics, including specialty; professional degree, such as MD or DO; employment status, such as private practice, partnership, or working as an employee for a larger parent company; the number of patient office visits by gender, race ethnicity, insurer, and age; the reason for visits from the patient and the provider perspective; and the number or percentage of preventive visits and visits due to injury. Surveys such as NAMCS provide important data to policymakers at the state and federal levels as they consider funding and regulatory legislation that impact providers and consumers.

Generate Statistical Reports for Financial Quality Improvement Measures

In the inpatient setting, one statistic that warrants attention from the finance office as well as the quality office is the **average length of stay (ALOS)**. Length of stay (LOS) refers to the number of days an inpatient remains in the hospital or care setting. This measure is not used in outpatient settings.

With the implementation of Medicare's **Prospective Payment System (PPS)** in the early 1980s, hospitals can no longer bill for services without constraint. Prior to PPS, physicians and hospitals made the decision on how long patients stayed in the hospital. In response to this system, the federal government through Medicare addressed concerns about increasing inpatient health care costs by establishing DRGs. DRGs outline what reimbursement hospitals receive for each service they provide. This holds the hospital responsible for cost control. To understand PPS, consider a patient was admitted for an appendectomy, a surgery performed to remove the appendix, as an example. Under PPS, the patient has a principal diagnosis of acute appendicitis and a principal procedure of appendectomy, uncomplicated. Uncomplicated indicates the patient was otherwise healthy. The hospital knows up front what it should receive reimbursement-wise for the patient. If the recommended payment includes consideration of a 3-day inpatient stay, and the hospital routinely keeps appendectomy patients for 4.5 days, the hospital still only receives reimbursement based on the 3 days allocated by the DRG assignment. Because an inpatient hospital day includes nursing care, laboratory services, pharmacy services, dietary services, and numerous supplies, hospitals that spend a full 1.5 days past the budget for the appendectomy patient quickly lose money. Multiply this by all the patients in hospital beds and you can see how quickly the length of stay becomes a financial issue.

You may work in a department that regularly calculates the ALOS for patient care units (PCUs), **service lines**, such as cardiology, internal medicine, or neurosurgery, physicians, or the entire hospital. The formula for calculating ALOS begins with the LOS. For example, consider a provider who admits about 10 patients a month to the hospital for diabetes-related complications. If in a month, the provider's 10 patients had LOS data as follows (in days) 3, 6, 2, 7, 9, 11, 4, 5, 5, 9, we can calculate the ALOS for the provider's patients that month by adding the total patient days together and dividing by the number of patients, which in this case is 10.

This month, the provider's patients' LOS calculates as:

3 + 6 + 2 + 7 + 9 + 11 + 4 + 5 + 5 + 9 = 61

His ALOS is 61 total patient days / 10 total patients = 6.1 days.

If the provider's ALOS of 6.1 days is higher than his colleagues who have similar patients, he should ask for data to investigate what practices his colleagues are using that helps get their patients home sooner. Clinicians and analysts rely on your skills to query the EHR and find the data under study.

While ALOS is not the only data that financial and clinical experts review, it is one of the more common. Learning to extract data from the EHR to analyze ALOS data also helps you to learn how to extract other data. The most important skill in this or other data extraction is your knowledge of the EHR, the data location, and how to query using predefined or ad hoc reports to get the data administrators need from patient records.

In the outpatient setting, statistical reports have a different focus, but the skills you need, such as knowledge of the EMR and the patient data it contains, remain the same.

Providers in outpatient settings may keep a closer eye on the financial impact of day-to-day decisions than they do in the hospital setting. This does not mean they care less about the impact in the hospital. In their private practices, providers often function as the clinician, **Chief Financial Officer (CFO)**, and quality control administrator. If you work as an EHR specialist in the outpatient setting, you can provide support to the clinical staff by learning the data and how best to query the patient records to extract necessary reports that support improvements to patient care or the financial bottom line.

In an outpatient setting, some of the reports you may need to query include the number of patients with various insurance coverage, the number or percentage of patients reporting to the facility for specific illnesses or procedures, or the number of patients in certain age groups. Statistics such as these can assist the clinical staff in planning for additional staff if the patient population is growing. These statistics can also identify if a specialty practitioner may be a necessary addition to the facility if they are seeing more patients with certain conditions. Statistics can provide the data to support acquiring equipment, such as an in-house ultrasound or glucometer for testing patients' blood glucose with a finger stick, or other equipment as patient patterns and populations indicate.

Regardless of the facility, you can provide answers to most data needs by learning the EHR or EMR system, communicating regularly with the clinical staff and others who use the data, and following or establishing a schedule to query for data that supports best practices in patient care and financial decisions.

Generate Aging Reports by Guarantor or Carrier

Many people have a hard time viewing facilities as businesses that require money and need to pursue patients who refuse to pay. However, facilities at every level must think like businesses in order to survive. The hospital, clinic, or physician office that ignores outstanding payments may find themselves in financial peril, with challenges to paying employees, upgrading outdated facilities, or paying bills.

Like most businesses, health care facilities have accounts receivable departments. **Accounts receivable** refers to the claims, or bills, the facility sends out for services they have a legal right to collect on. In other words, it is money the facility expects to receive for goods and services the patient has already received. In health care, this is complex for a number of reasons.

In retail, when you purchase a suit, the full price that is set by the seller is what you pay. In health care, an office visit for a Medicare patient is likely billed at a different rate than the same office visit for a commercial or private insurance patient. This is because of negotiated or contracted rates, meaning insurers and providers negotiate the price of services on a regular basis. Providers agree to only charge patients with certain insurance coverage a specific price, which can differ from other insurance carriers.

The patient's expected contribution is also part of negotiating the price of services. It specifies the maximum amount the provider can charge for the service. Consider a routine office visit that is problem-focused and medically simple where the provider receives a reimbursement payment of $55 from the insurer. The **commercial insurer** and provider contractually agree that for a routine office visit the provider receives a reimbursement payment of $55 from the insurer, and that the patient pays a $20 **copayment**. If the provider has the set price for this routine visit at $125, she cannot bill the patient for the difference. These negotiations go on among insurers and providers across the country. Patients without insurance often fare the worst. They pay the full price for the same service because they have no insurance company negotiating for them toward a reduced rate. Medicare may contract to pay $45 and Medicaid may only agree to pay $25 – all for the same service.

Provider Service	Provider Price	Contractual Rate Reimbursed by Insurer			Patient Copay
		Commercial Insurance #1	Medicare	Medicaid	
Routine Office Visit	$125	$55	$45	$25	$20
Moderately Complex Office Visit	$175	$75	$65	$37	$20

This chart is for illustration purposes only. It should not be viewed as data on actual rates.

In the hospital setting, the practice of creating and reviewing reports on outstanding accounts is an established, formal work assignment within a single department. This department, usually the finance department, focuses on the financial matters of the hospital. Regular reporting is performed here and members of the senior leadership team, such as the CFO and **Chief Executive Officer (CEO)**, review the reports to ensure the facility's financial health remains stable.

For smaller outpatient settings, determining who owes money and when they will pay is critical, as there is often less wiggle room to accommodate late payments or delinquent accounts than in a larger facility. As an EHR specialist, you can make a difference by staying up to date with these reports. Understanding the characteristics of insurers and knowing how to query the EMR or other software to extract billing and reimbursement information by patient, insurer, or other contributes to the facility's financial health.

Generate Financial Analysis Reports by Provider, Diagnosis, or Procedure

Another aspect in the evaluation of the financial health of a facility is the difference between various providers, diagnoses, and procedures.

For example, to determine if a surgeon is performing cardiac surgery correctly, you first need to pull data on all patients who have undergone the same surgery in your facility. Next, separate the data by surgeon and evaluate the patients' health status by surgeon. This needs to include a review of patients who have **complications**, **comorbidities**, or other conditions that are separate, but contribute to a patient's health and probable prognosis. As this example illustrates, it is important to use data to make decisions. It is necessary to report on data at this finite level of detail in facilities every day to answer important financial questions. These financial questions include: which providers positively contribute to the facility's financial health and which do not; which admissions based on principal diagnosis are most financially lucrative and which are not; and which procedures are financially beneficial to the organization and which are not? As an EHR specialist, you can help your facility make important decisions by making information available in reports and data tables to illustrate the facts.

In outpatient settings, carefully prepare reports on insurance carriers who support the most patients and the procedures and diagnoses that generate the most revenue. This information proves useful for the physicians to make decisions. Expanding the patient population has implications depending on the insurance distribution. For example, a commercial insurer may reimburse at a higher level than a government insurer. Advertising for new patients may be an option for increasing the patient population, but knowing what kinds of patients you can manage from a financial perspective is important, too. Providers' practice patterns may also prove to be lucrative or money-losers. Knowing which procedures fall into either category assists the physicians in making decisions that impact everyone in the facility, including patients and employees. For example, suppose the removal of skin lesions is a normal procedure in a facility. In a general office setting, this procedure may take more time than services, such as physicals, visits for colds, and care for chronic diseases common among the elderly population. A query of the patients who had skin lesion removal procedures last year and a comparison of the reimbursement for this against the reimbursement for the other standard office visits may show there is little difference. The next step is to review the scheduling for this procedure. Access the practice management software and query the database to see if scheduling skin lesion procedures impacts the number of other visits. A simple data analysis like this might show that although the procedures generate similar revenue, the physician time spent on a skin lesion procedure for a single patient could accommodate two patients with more standard visits, potentially doubling the reimbursement for that time period.

There is no way to anticipate the number and type of queries to patient and financial data that you may perform in either the inpatient or outpatient setting. If you know the EHR or EMR system and are familiar with the data that exists within it and any related systems, you will be a valuable asset to your facility and the patients you serve.

Summary

As an EHR specialist, you provide vital support to a facility when you learn the reporting needs of your facility and when you are familiar with the data.

QI measures, whether internal or mandated from external agencies, rely on accurate recording and reporting of data. To provide accurate and timely reports, learn the inpatient and outpatient statistics that are commonly collected and options for collecting and storing data.

Financial concerns are always an issue. As an EHR specialist, your proactive approach to evaluating and reporting on critical financial data serves your facility and patients. Understanding the various insurer requirements and contracts can help determine which data to query, and knowing how to evaluate the financial impact by provider, diagnosis, or procedure provides your facility with the information it needs to remain financially stable.

Drill Questions

1. Comparing quality data from a facility against data provided by external agencies or an internal goal is called which of the following?

   A. Data quality assessment
   B. Benchmarking
   C. Continuous QI
   D. Accreditation

2. When an EHR specialist reviewed hospital data, she found that when one provider admits patients, the facility's revenues increased, and when another provider admits patients, revenues declined. After figuring out both providers practice internal medicine and admit the same type of patients, the EHR specialist should look at which of the following data first?

   A. Total inpatient service days
   B. Occupancy rate
   C. Average length of stay
   D. Mortality rate

3. Accounts receivable is

   A. the number of patient accounts an EHR specialist can expect to add in a future, defined period.
   B. the number of vendor accounts the hospital has active and open.
   C. the amount the hospital owes to an external business for goods and services already received.
   D. the amount due to the hospital for goods and services already provided.

4. If an EHR specialist works in a provider's office, he may need to provide data in response to which of the following?

   A. CMS CoPs site survey
   B. A Joint Commission inquiry on aspirin for patients who had a heart attack
   C. NAMCS
   D. A state department of health inquiry on the physical structure of the practice

5. A patient is covered by commercial insurance, while her neighbor has no insurance. When the patient's neighbor went to her provider's office for a chest cold, she was billed $137.50 for the visit and a strep test. The insured patient wonders why her explanation of benefits only shows a payment of $42 for her office visit, even though they saw the same provider. Which of the following explains the cost difference?

   A. Laboratory tests are expensive and often cost more than the provider's time.
   B. The bill was sent in error and the patient's neighbor will receive a new one.
   C. Insurance companies negotiate discounted rates that are generally lower than the actual price set by the provider's office.
   D. Self-pay patients need to negotiate the price for services when scheduling appointments.

6. Which of the following results in a hospital financial inquiry on patients who receive treatment for the same illness or injury?

   A. Higher length of stay than average
   B. Morbidity
   C. Lower length of stay than average
   D. Mortality

7. PPS helps control costs through which of the following practices?

   A. Relying on families to care for patients who are discharged early
   B. Relying on private providers to continue the care that began in the hospital once the patient is discharged
   C. Paying every inpatient stay at the same level and requiring hospitals to submit justification for any increase in payment
   D. Predefining the payment for services based on principal diagnosis

8. The need for EHR specialists who can query, analyze, and report on health data is likely to do which of the following?

   A. Diminish as computer technology replaces human work
   B. Increase as legal and regulatory pressures continue to place demands on facilities
   C. Level out and stay the same
   D. Vary between facilities with some needing more analysis and others needing less

9. A hospital financial director needs information on cost controls. The CFO believes that one or two providers are driving up costs due to their patterns of practice. However, the CEO believes the cost is likely due to having too many medical patients and not enough surgical patients. Which of the following reports should return the data both senior leaders need confirm or correct their assumptions?

    A. Daily census by PCU and provider

    B. ALOS report by provider and service line

    C. Mortality report by service line and PCU

    D. Morbidity report by provider and service line

Drill Answers

1. Comparing quality data from a facility against data provided by external agencies or an internal goal is called which of the following?

   A. Data quality assessment
   B. Benchmarking
   C. Continuous QI
   D. Accreditation

   Benchmarking is the process by which a facility compares itself to other facilities or set goals or metrics. Data quality assessment is by definition, not comparison. Continuous QI is an internal QI process. It may include benchmarking as one of the steps toward quality. Accreditation is the evaluation by an external agency or facility based on predetermined standards.

2. When an EHR specialist reviewed hospital data, she found that when one provider admits patients, the facility's revenues increased, and when another provider admits patients, revenues declined. After figuring out both providers practice internal medicine and admit the same type of patients, the EHR specialist should look at which of the following data first?

   A. Total inpatient service days
   B. Occupancy rate
   C. Average length of stay
   D. Mortality rate

   Under PPS, hospitals receive reimbursement based on predetermined rates. A longer length of stay without documentation of acceptable reasons to justify a higher reimbursement costs the hospital money. Total inpatient service days provide the number of patients in the patient care unit or hospital. Occupancy rate provides the percentage of licensed beds that are filled with a patient. Mortality rate, or death rate, is important, but not in determining revenue differences.

3. Accounts receivable is

   A. the number of patient accounts an EHR specialist can expect to add in a future, defined period.
   B. the number of vendor accounts the hospital has active and open.
   C. the amount the hospital owes to an external business for goods and services already received.
   D. the amount due to the hospital for goods and services already provided.

   Accounts receivable is the amount due to the hospital for goods and services already provided. It represents the amount of money the facility legally is entitled to receive based on the provision of services.

4. If an EHR specialist works in a provider's office, he may need to provide data in response to which of the following?

    A. CMS CoPs site survey
    B. A Joint Commission inquiry on aspirin for patients who had a heart attack
    C. NAMCS
    D. A state department of health inquiry on the physical structure of the practice

NAMCS is a national survey that collects data on ambulatory medical care. CMS does not require provider offices to abide by CoPs. Data for a Joint Commission inquiry on aspirin for patients who had a heart attack is not found in a provider's office. State health departments may have space requirements, but this would not require a query of the patient database.

5. A patient is covered by commercial insurance, while her neighbor has no insurance. When the patient's neighbor went to her provider's office for a chest cold, she was billed $137.50 for the visit and a strep test. The insured patient wonders why her explanation of benefits only shows a payment of $42 for her office visit, even though they saw the same provider. Which of the following explains the cost difference?

    A. Laboratory tests are expensive and often cost more than the provider's time.
    B. The bill was sent in error and the patient's neighbor will receive a new one.
    C. Insurance companies negotiate discounted rates that are generally lower than the actual price set by the provider's office.
    D. Self-pay patients need to negotiate the price for services when scheduling appointments.

One of the benefits of a patient having insurance is that the insurance company negotiates how much it will pay for services, so the patient does not have to pay the full asking price the office sets, whereas self-pay patients have to pay the full asking price. Laboratory tests are expensive and often cost more than the provider's time is not a viable explanation for the cost difference. The bill was sent in error and the patient's neighbor will receive a new one is not a likely explanation for the cost difference. While patients may negotiate the payment terms, such as paying in installments or deferring the bill, they generally have no negotiating power when it comes to price.

6. Which of the following results in a hospital financial inquiry on patients who receive treatment for the same illness or injury?

    A. Higher length of stay than average
    B. Morbidity
    C. Lower length of stay than average
    D. Mortality

    Under PPS, hospitals are reimbursed at set rates. Keeping a patient in-house longer than approved costs the hospital money and discharging a patient sooner than approved saves the hospital money. Morbidity refers to the presence of disease. Mortality refers to death.

7. PPS helps control costs through which of the following practices?

    A. Relying on families to care for patients who are discharged early
    B. Relying on private providers to continue the care that began in the hospital once the patient is discharged
    C. Paying every inpatient stay at the same level and requiring hospitals to submit justification for any increase in payment
    D. Predefining the payment for services based on principal diagnosis

    The purpose of PPS is to hold hospitals accountable for the care they provide by giving a set amount of money that the hospital must manage effectively and efficiently. Relying on families to care for patients who are discharged early is not part of the PPS plan for decreasing costs – neither is relying on private providers to continue the care that began in the hospital once the patient is discharged. Paying every inpatient stay at the same level and requiring hospitals to submit justification for any increase in payment is also not part of the PPS plan for decreasing costs.

8. The need for EHR specialists who can query, analyze, and report on health data is likely to do which of the following?

    A. Diminish as computer technology replaces human work
    B. Increase as legal and regulatory pressures continue to place demands on facilities
    C. Level out and stay the same
    D. Vary between facilities with some needing more analysis and others needing less

Governmental and regulatory agencies continue to expand demands for data and seek justification for reimbursement that requires more and more data. While some work may be replaced by computers, it is not likely that computers will replace EHR specialists. Given past patterns, the need for EHR specialists will not level out and stay the same. Regulatory and government requirements generally apply across all facilities. Therefore, it is not likely to vary between facilities with some needing more analysis and others needing less.

9. A hospital financial director needs information on cost controls. The CFO believes that one or two providers are driving up costs due to their patterns of practice. However, the CEO believes the cost is likely due to having too many medical patients and not enough surgical patients. Which of the following reports should return the data both senior leaders need confirm or correct their assumptions?

    A. Daily census by PCU and provider
    B. ALOS report by provider and service line
    C. Mortality report by service line and PCU
    D. Morbidity report by provider and service line

A report on ALOS by provider and service line should answer both the CEO's and CFO's questions. The daily consensus, the mortality report, and the morbidity report would not give the CEO or CFO the information they need.

Terms and Definitions

Accounts receivable – Patient bills for services that have already been provided that legally are due to a facility

Autopsy rates – The percent of autopsies performed on patients who die in the hospital; reasons for not performing an autopsy in the hospital may include legal inquiry or family preference

Average length of stay (ALOS) – The total number of patient days in a period divided by the number of patients; for example, the ALOS for cardiology services in February was 6.1 days

Benchmarks – Goals or metrics a facility wants to meet; for example, if the industry standard is 90% of patients should have advance directives entered into their patient record within 24 hr of admission, and a hospital was only meeting this for 45% of the patients, they would use the external benchmark of 90% as a goal and track performance toward that goal by month or quarter

Centers for Disease Control and Prevention (CDC) – A division of the Department of Health and Human Services

Chief executive officer (CEO) – Leader of a facility who reports to the Board of Directors

Chief financial officer (CFO) – Leader who oversees all financial and fiscal decisions and issues for a facility; generally reports to the CEO

Commercial insurers – Private, non-government insurers; these are often the insurance options available through employers

Comorbidity – Disease that exists at the same time as a primary disease that a patient is being treated for at that time; for example, a patient who has cancer is receiving cancer-specific treatment and is also a diabetic – diabetes mellitus would be considered the comorbid condition

Complications – Unexpected events or circumstances that happen to a patient during the course of his care; hospital-acquired infections, such as those involving MRSA, are considered to be complications, as are reactions to medications or an adverse response to any treatment

Copayment – Money the patient must pay toward the bill as contracted between the insurer and provider; amounts range from $5 to $50, and $75 for emergency room and specialist visits; provider's office visits are often in the $10 to $35 range

Daily census – The count of how many patients are in beds by patient care unit for an inpatient facility

Department of Health and Human Services (HHS) – Principle agency for protecting Americans' health

Institute of Medicine (IOM) – Non-governmental, independent, and nonprofit organization that provides unbiased, expert advice to governmental and private decision-makers, as well as the public

Morbidity – Refers to disease

Mortality (death) rate – The percentage of all discharged patients who are discharged due to death within a prescribed period; for example, if a hospital has discharged 30 patients in a month, and of those 5 were deaths, the mortality rate for the month would be expressed as 5/30 or 16.7%

National Ambulatory Medical Care Survey (NAMCS) – Collects data on ambulatory medical care provided in the U.S.; the data is collected from visits to office-based providers who provide direct patient care

National Center for Health Statistics (NCHS) – Nation's primary statistics organization; it works to compile, analyze, and disseminate information on the nation's health to influence and guide health policy and practice in a manner that best serves the population

National Hospital Inpatient Quality Measures – A set of specific data that hospitals must collect and report to CMS and the Joint Commission to document quality patient care

Occupancy rate – The percentage of licensed beds in a hospital that have a patient assigned to them, and thus are generating revenue

Patient care unit (PCU) – For the purpose of census data, a PCU has a defined number of beds and is staff assigned; also called floors, units, or wards

Prospective Payment System (PPS) – System initially implemented by Medicare in the early 1980s that replaced fee-for-service payments for the provision of health services with predetermined payments based on the principal diagnosis of the patient

Service lines – Groups of patient services by specialty; hospitals define these individually, and they vary by facility with some similarities, such as obstetrics; examples include cardiology, neurology, thoracic surgery, general surgery, and gynecology; some facilities choose to combine similar or related lines, such as obstetrics and neonatology, obstetrics and gynecology, and cardio-thoracic surgery; they are useful for compiling financial, compliance, and other in-house reports

Total inpatient service days – The number of inpatients receiving care each day summed for the days in the period under study; for example, if you are reviewing the total inpatient service days for the month of September, which has 30 days, add the patients for Sept 1 (125), Sept 2 (119), and so on; the total is the sum of all patients per day

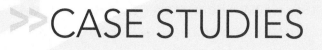

Quick Access to Patient Information

Jill Smith is a patient lying on a bed in an emergency department bay. She is confused and groggy from a head injury. Susan, an emergency department nurse, and Fran, the unit's EHR specialist, are in the room with her. Susan introduces herself and asks Jill if she can tell her what happened.

Jill is unable to recall the incident because she is still groggy, so Susan addresses Marti, Jill's sister, about what happened.

"We were walking downtown, and I'm not exactly sure what happened," Marti says. "But I was walking in front of her, and I turned just as Jill was falling off the sidewalk. She hit her head pretty hard."

"It would be helpful if we had her past medical history. Do you happen to know how we can get in touch with her primary care provider?" Susan asks.

"I know she sees Dr. Richard Birks. Here's the insurance card. The doctor's office phone number is on there," Marti says.

Susan hands the insurance card to Fran, who then starts to type the information into the COW.

"Great. Once Fran gets her entered into our system, she will call and get her medical information sent over," Susan says to Marti.

"Marti?" Jill says.

"I'm here, Jill," Marti says.

"Hello, my name is Susan, I'm the nurse. Your sister tells me you fell and hit your head. Do you know where you are?"

"Hospital?" Jill says.

"Yes, that's right. Do you think you can answer a couple of questions for Fran?" Susan asks. "Fran is the unit's EHR specialist. She manages the administrative duties. I'm going to meet with the doctor, and then I'll come back to take care of your head."

Once Jill nods yes, Fran moves the COW and begins to ask her questions.

"Can you give me your full name?"

"Jill Anne Smith."

As Jill is answering, Fran is verifying the information matches the insurance card.

Jill says her head hurts, so Marti begins answering the questions.

"Her address is 555 Hillside Avenue, San Diego, California. The zip code is 90203."

"Date of birth?"

At this point, Jill starts to answer.

"March 19, 1943."

"Marital status?"

"Widowed."

"Okay, I also need to list next of kin or an emergency contact. Should I go ahead and list your sister?"

Jill nods yes.

"Great. I have your insurance card here already, so we're almost done with this part. But I do still have a couple more questions. Do you have any allergies to medication?"

Jill doesn't respond, so Marti answers that Jill is allergic to aspirin.

"Okay, any other allergies or medication that you have been advised to avoid?" Fran asks. "The nurse will ask you these questions again, but we try to document as much of this up front as possible."

Jill shakes her head no.

"How are we doing here?" Susan asks Fran as she re-enters the room.

"Just getting allergy information."

"Do you take any prescription medication?" Fran asks Jill.

"I take a daily multivitamin, but nothing else."

Fran finishes entering the data into the computer and hits enter to print a patient armband. She hands the armband to Susan.

"Okay, please confirm for me your name and your date of birth. I'll need your left arm, please," Susan says to Jill.

Jill extends her left arm toward Susan and says, "Jill Anne Smith, March 19, 1943."

"Terrific. Here you go. The doctor should be in to see you shortly," Susan says as she fastens the armband, which has a visible barcode printed on it, to Jill's arm.

"I still have such a headache," Jill says.

"We can't give you anything until we get some information from your doctor and our doctor examines you."

Fran clicks and types on the keyboard.

"Looks like the eFax just came through," Fran says. "I'll print it out and put it with the intake form so the doctor has it when he is ready to examine her."

"I'll make a note in your chart about your headache – it won't be long 'til the doctor sees you," Susan says.

Susan leaves Jill's room, taking the COW with her.

Dr. Chen, who is holding a tablet PC and a stylus, walks into where Jill's bed is in the emergency department bay.

"Hello, Ms. Smith, I'm Dr. Chen. Your doctor's office faxed us your past medical history and you seem to be pretty healthy," he says. "I see you had knee surgery 2 years ago with good results and a hysterectomy 10 years ago, but other than that, you're in good shape, even after your fall."

"I guess so, but my head sure hurts. Can you give me anything for this pain?" Jill asks.

"Yes. I can prescribe acetaminophen, which is a non-aspirin pain reliever, and that should give you some relief. I'll get Fran to coach me here. We're using a new, computerized system to prescribe medication, so we've got help down here while we all get used to this new system."

Dr. Chen holds out the tablet PC and Fran shows him how to enter the order into the tablet.

"The hospital is now using a Computerized Provider Order Entry or CPOE system for all prescriptions and other orders. It is faster, safer, and more reliable than paper prescriptions. Once Dr. Chen hit the enter button on the screen, the order was sent to the pharmacy, and they fill it and send it back up here for you," Fran says.

"With Fran's help, I have entered the order, so they should be able to get that for you while we're wrapping up this paperwork so you can get out of here," Dr. Chen says.

"Thank you, both," Jill says.

Susan returns to the room with the COW, a cup of water, discharge papers, and a pill blister pack with a barcode on the back.

"Hello again, I see that Dr. Chen prescribed some acetaminophen for your headache and signed for your discharge instructions so we can get you out of here. First, let's get you this pain medication. Can you give me your arm?" Susan asks.

Jill raises her arm toward Susan, revealing the armband and barcode.

"Okay, now again, can you confirm your name and date of birth?" Susan asks.

"Jill Anne Smith, March 19, 1943."

Susan picks up the barcode scanner from the COW and scans Jill's armband. The barcode scanner beeps once. Susan lays the barcode scanner down and picks up the small cup of water and hands it to Jill. Susan then picks up the sealed packet of medication from a drawer on the COW and scans the barcode on the back of the packet with the barcode scanner. After it beeps once, Susan hits the enter button on the keyboard to capture the data.

"Great. There's your water and here's your pills," Susan says as she peels the back off the pill packet and drops two pills into Jill's open hand without touching the pills.

"Thank you," Jill says, popping the pills into her mouth.

"Now, let's go over your discharge instructions. If after you get home you begin to experience severe dizziness, your headache gets worse, or you begin to have vision problems, you need to call us or come back in to be seen," Susan says.

"Okay," Jill says, nodding her head.

"Alright then, here's your copy of the discharge instructions, along with the phone number here if you need to call us. The instructions we just covered and what to do if you start to feel worse are listed as well," Susan says as she picks up the discharge paper from the COW and hands Jill the paper.

"Great, thank you," Jill says.

Susan hands Jill an electronic signature pad with a plastic pen attached.

"Now, I just need your signature here, confirming you have received and understand the discharge instructions, and you're good to go," Susan says.

1. Which of the following parts of Jill's health record carries information regarding her potential treatment and recovery?

    A. Insurance information
    B. Past medical history
    C. Patient information sheet
    D. Consents and acknowledgements

2. If Dr. Chen orders a pain pill that contains aspirin using the EHR system's CPOE, which of the following prevents Jill from receiving the medication?

    A. Quality assurance checks in the pharmacy
    B. The EHR clinical decision support tool
    C. The nurse who remembers Jill's aspirin allergy
    D. The provider who considers Jill's faxed medical data

3. Now that Jill is discharged from the emergency department, the hospital should do which of the following with the fax it received from Jill's provider's office?

    A. Mail the document back to Jill.
    B. File the document in a traditional paper-based medical record folder.
    C. Mail the document back to Jill's provider.
    D. Scan the document into Jill's record in the EHR system.

4. Six months later, an emergency department pharmacy issue requires all medications dispensed to patients in the emergency department to be reviewed. Which of the following describes how the pharmacy analyst should track who dispensed medication to patients during that time period?

   A. Review the pharmacy records for a list of prescribing providers for that period.
   B. Interview emergency department personnel to document what they recall for the time period.
   C. Review data captured from the barcode scans of the medications and the patient armbands.
   D. Audit emergency department records for the time period to document providers who prescribed medications.

5. Several weeks later, Marti stops by the emergency department because Jill asked her to pick up a copy of her emergency department visit record so she can populate her personal health record. Which of the following is the correct response from the records clerk?

   A. "Sure! Because you were here with your sister, this is not a problem. I'll get that for you right away."
   B. "I'm sorry, I can't release it to you in person, but I can have it sent to you as long as you live with your sister."
   C. "I'm sorry, I can't release your sister's records without her documented permission."
   D. "If you remember the name of the nurse who treated your sister, he or she may remember you and authorize us to release it to you."

Quick Access to Patient Information: Answers

1. Which of the following parts of Jill's health record carries information regarding her potential treatment and recovery?

   A. Insurance information
   B. Past medical history
   C. Patient information sheet
   D. Consents and acknowledgements

   Past medical history alerts the treating provider to the patient's prior and existing medical conditions, medications, medication allergies, and other relevant issues that may affect the patient's treatment and recovery. Insurance information, the patient information sheet, and consents and acknowledgements have no impact on the patient's treatment and recovery.

2. If Dr. Chen orders a pain pill that contains aspirin using the EHR system's CPOE, which of the following prevents Jill from receiving the medication?

   A. Quality assurance checks in the pharmacy
   B. The EHR clinical decision support tool
   C. The nurse who remembers Jill's aspirin allergy
   D. The provider who considers Jill's faxed medical data

   Clinical decision support provides patient-specific information to enhance health-related decisions at the point of care. This includes medication-allergy checking/alerts, dosage guidance, duplicate therapy checking/alerts, and medication–medication interaction checking/alerts.

3. Now that Jill is discharged from the emergency department, the hospital should do which of the following with the fax it received from Jill's provider's office?

    A. Mail the document back to Jill.
    B. File the document in a traditional paper-based medical record folder.
    C. Mail the document back to Jill's provider.
    D. Scan the document into Jill's record in the EHR system.

Scanning paper documents into a facility's EHR software is the best way to make non-digital information available in a digital or electronic format. Once the document is scanned into the EHR system, the hard copy must be shredded for confidentially purposes. Medical record documents are not sent to patients unless specifically requested. Filing the document in a traditional paper-based medical record folder is not applicable because the hospital has an EHR system. Mailing the document back to Jill's provider is not applicable because the provider has the original copy.

4. Six months later, an emergency department pharmacy issue requires all medications dispensed to patients in the emergency department to be reviewed. Which of the following describes how the pharmacy analyst should track who dispensed medication to patients during that time period?

    A. Review the pharmacy records for a list of prescribing providers for that period.
    B. Interview emergency department personnel to document what they recall for the time period.
    C. Review data captured from the barcode scans of the medications and the patient armbands.
    D. Audit emergency department records for the time period to document providers who prescribed medications.

Barcode technology records the patient's name, ID, and other identifying information, along with the name of the attending physician in the EHR system. This allows the analyst to obtain information about the medications the pharmacy dispenses to patients. Therefore, a list of providers is not sufficient information. The analyst should not interview emergency department personnel to document what they recall, nor should the analyst audit emergency department records for the time period to document providers who prescribed medications because they are not efficient or accurate methods for obtaining this data.

5. Several weeks later, Marti stops by the emergency department because Jill asked her to pick up a copy of her emergency department visit record so she can populate her personal health record. Which of the following is the correct response from the records clerk?

    A. "Sure! Because you were here with your sister, this is not a problem. I'll get that for you right away."

    B. "I'm sorry, I can't release it to you in person, but I can have it sent to you as long as you live with your sister."

    C. "I'm sorry, I can't release your sister's records without her documented permission."

    D. "If you remember the name of the nurse who treated your sister, he or she may remember you and authorize us to release it to you."

Family members cannot obtain medical record information for a family member without the patient's authorization. Marti cannot request her sister's health care information.

Technology in the Outpatient Setting

Janet, the office manager, and Karen, the EHR specialist, are sitting at a computer at the reception desk in a provider's office and talking about how the practice uses its EHR system.

"We're glad to have you, Karen. This practice keeps getting busier and busier," Janet says. "We need someone with expertise in using and maintaining our electronic health records."

"Thanks. I'm a little nervous, but happy to be here!" Karen says.

"The first thing we do in the morning is to run a report for the scheduled patient visits by provider so the doctors and Leila, the nurse practitioner, have some idea who they are seeing and what the day's schedule looks like," Janet says. "I'm going to pull Dr. Johnson's patients to show you how we do it. You can then pull Dr. Stone's and Leila's patients."

"Once the computer is on, log on with your username and password, then you click to open Practice Charts, that's our EHR system, and click on this button to find the reports we use. Once you're in the Reports section, click on the icon that says Daily Patient Schedules," Janet says, clicking three times on the computer screen.

"Now, click here and select one of the providers. I'm going to choose Dr. Johnson," she says, clicking two more times.

"I will select a date here and then select print. It will default to the printer up here and will always print two copies. One is for us here at the front desk, and one is for each of the doctor's offices so they don't have to come up here to find the schedule," Janet says.

Karen walks over to the printer to grab the pieces of paper, hands them to Janet, and says, "Here you go."

"Good. Now, we have clipboards where we place these reports. There are two for each provider – one for his office and one for here at the front desk. There is a blue plastic sheet that stays on each clipboard, and the patient list goes under that plastic," Janet says, picking up the two clipboards with blue plastic sheets on them. "So, if people are standing nearby, they can't read the patient's names from the list – that's a privacy issue and it's important."

"Gotcha," Karen says.

"Okay, it's your turn. I'm going to log out. As you know, that's important. Never leave your computer on and logged in with your username and password. That's a privacy and security issue for our patients, but it also protects you. We run user activity reports so anytime there is a question about who accessed a patient record, we have the date, time, and user ID of the person who logged into the record. Go ahead and log in," Janet says, getting up from the chair and letting Karen sit down at the computer.

"Yes, in my last position, I was in charge of the audit reporting that checked all the system activity," Karen says, logging into the computer.

With Janet's help, Karen creates a report and puts the printouts under the blue sheets on the appropriate clip boards.

"Perfect!" Janet says. "Now let's check the wireless connections and get the exam rooms opened and ready. The doctors will be in soon from hospital rounds and we want to make sure they can access the system when they log in."

Karen stands up and picks up the provider's half of the clipboards and follows Janet to one of the treatment rooms. In the room, they meet Leila.

"Hi, I'm Leila, the nurse practitioner. Here's what we do after we see the patient. We'll mark the appropriate codes in the computer and print it. It prints at the patient check-out area."

Karen nods her head in agreement.

"You'll check the E&M code to make sure that it fits the visit scheduled. You know, if the visit is brief, limited, or extended," Janet says. "Look to see that the examination is checked. This document shows how many body systems the provider examined on the patient. As you can imagine, this can range from one for a simple sinus infection to a complete exam for patients with more complex issues."

"You'll also want to check to see that the code accurately represents whether it's a new patient or an established patient and how much time the provider spent. Most of the time these are correct, but we want to provide a second review for accuracy," Leila says.

"I know it's important for the code to reflect the history, physical exam, the medical decision making, and time spent with the patient," Karen says, counting off each one on her hand.

"That's right – the reimbursement depends on an accurate capture of the time each clinician spends with the patient. With your training and experience in coding and billing, I'm sure you'll do just fine," Janet says. "Let's go find Dr. Stone and introduce you."

Karen and Janet walk back to the reception area to meet Dr. Stone, who is standing behind the desk, looking over her diabetes study.

"You remember Karen, Dr. Stone, from her interview?" Janet asks. "I think Karen is off to a good start this morning."

"Good morning, Karen, welcome!" Dr. Stone says. "I have something new here that we'll need your help on."

"Great," Karen replies.

"The hospital administrators are interested in coordinating better care for diabetic patients and are inviting providers' offices to participate in a diabetes registry. This will help us track the disease and the treatments, as well as provide a database of patients who have diabetes in the region," Dr. Stone says. "Then, we can better track trends and patterns. Hopefully it will help us better serve our diabetic patients."

"That sounds like the cancer registry we had at the hospital I worked at a couple of years ago," Karen says.

"Yes, it's very similar. The only difference is that this is based on the entire population in this area and not just a single facility. It will serve many of the same purposes. Here's the information from the Diabetes Project at the hospital," Dr. Stone says, handing the papers to Karen. "It explains what they are hoping to collect, and I think our EHR system will make this a simple job on our end."

"We'll work on pulling together an initial report of active patients today and can move on to archived patients later," Janet says.

Karen nods in agreement.

"Thanks!" Dr. Stone says. "Looking forward to your results."

"Now, let's take care of these patients," Janet says, pointing to the number system on the wall. "They take numbers when they come in, so instead of a sign-in sheet, we can call them by number and then deal with each patient in a private manner here at the desk. Go ahead and call patient number one."

Karen looks out into the waiting room and asks, "May I have patient number one come to the front desk?"

Mrs. Simpson stands up and walks to the front desk and hands Karen a plastic square with a large, black #1 on it.

"Good morning. May I please have your name?" Karen asks.

"Mrs. Barbara Simpson. I have an 8 o'clock appointment with Dr. Stone."

"Yes, you're right here," Karen says, making a check mark beside her name on the clipboard. "I'll just verify your insurance information and then I can take you to the exam room."

Mrs. Simpson hands Karen her insurance card.

"Has anything changed with your insurance since your last visit, Mrs. Simpson?" Karen asks.

"No, I'm still on Medicare and even have the same insurance card."

Karen picks up the insurance card and swipes it through a small scanner. Once she scans and swipes it on both sides, she clicks the mouse several times and hands the card back to Mrs. Simpson.

"Okay, you're good to go. Come on back, and Dr. Stone will see you soon," Karen says.

"Okay, good. Thank you."

1. The data the practice collects from patient records for the regional diabetes registry can be used in a public report only after which of the following?

   A. Patients sign a ROI form, allowing their data to be included in the report.
   B. The data is de-identified so no patient demographic information can be extracted from the report.
   C. A disclaimer is posted on the report, noting the facility followed HIPAA privacy regulations during data collection.
   D. Patients submit a consent form to the CDC, allowing information to be used for statistical purposes only.

2. Which of the following specifically captures and bills for the time a provider spends with a patient?

   A. HCPCS
   B. ICD-10-CM
   C. E&M
   D. CPT

3. When Janet reminded Karen to always log off the computer when she was not using it, she mentioned user activity reports. As they relate to compliance with HIPAA regulations, these reports are also called which of the following?

    A. Productivity reports
    B. Audit trail reports
    C. Meaningful Use Measures reports
    D. Practice management reports

4. The facility in this scenario uses a number system for patient check-in. Some practices prefer this method for which of the following reasons?

    A. The staff avoids mispronouncing patients' names.
    B. The process is more efficient than a registration workflow.
    C. It protects patients' privacy.
    D. Sign-in sheets make unreliable permanent records.

5. After seeing Mrs. Simpson, Dr. Stone refers her to a specialist. Which of the following helps make the necessary referral paperwork simple and quick at check-out?

    A. Insurance verification process
    B. Online appointment scheduling
    C. Health maintenance reminders
    D. Customized templates

6. An older adult patient seen that day reports his medical history includes "sugar" on both sides of his family. While Karen knows this refers to diabetes mellitus, she also realizes it is important for providers to document precisely in the EHR. Which of the following helps standardize data elements and descriptions of medical terms in the EHR?

    A. SNOMED-CT
    B. ICD-10-CM
    C. CPT-4
    D. HCPCS

7. A transport ambulance service the facility partially owns brought in one of the patients that day. The coder was unable to assign a CPT code for the service. Which of the following actions should the coder perform to obtain reimbursement?

    A. Bill the patient directly for the ambulance transport.
    B. Write off the charges because the facility partially owns the ambulance.
    C. Submit a claim form with a HCPCS Level II code.
    D. Assign a CPT code that resembles a nonemergency ambulance transport.

Technology in the Outpatient Setting: Answers

1. The data the practice collects from patient records for the regional diabetes registry can be used in a public report only after which of the following?

    A. Patients sign a ROI form, allowing their data to be included in the report.
    B. **The data is de-identified so no patient demographic information can be extracted from the report.**
    C. A disclaimer is posted on the report, noting the facility followed HIPAA privacy regulations during data collection.
    D. Patients submit a consent form to the CDC, allowing information to be used for statistical purposes only.

    Public reporting commonly uses de-identified data. Data cannot be released to the public with identifiable information. Data that will be de-identified prior to use does not require specific patient authorization. A disclaimer does not waive responsibility to adhere to HIPAA laws. The CDC does not require patients to submit a consent form for statistical diabetes data.

2. Which of the following specifically captures and bills for the time a provider spends with a patient?

    A. HCPCS
    B. ICD-10-CM
    C. **E&M**
    D. CPT

    CPT E&M codes capture the amount and the intensity of time the provider spends with the patient. HCPCS codes capture supplies and non-provider services that are not captured with CPT codes. ICD-10-CM codes capture patient diagnoses. CPT codes capture all provider, diagnostic, and therapeutic services.

3. When Janet reminded Karen to always log off the computer when she was not using it, she mentioned user activity reports. As they relate to compliance with HIPAA regulations, these reports are also called which of the following?

    A. Productivity reports
    B. Audit trail reports
    C. Meaningful Use Measures reports
    D. Practice management reports

Audit trail reports track user activity, time of log in and log out, and the areas accessed. Productivity reports are not a concern in regard to HIPAA regulations. Meaningful Use Measures reports are used to report health information to CMS and to track key clinical indicators. Practice management reports may include a section on audit trails, but are not specific to this issue.

4. The facility in this scenario uses a number system for patient check-in. Some practices prefer this method for which of the following reasons?

    A. The staff avoids mispronouncing patients' names.
    B. The process is more efficient than a registration workflow.
    C. It protects patients' privacy.
    D. Sign-in sheets make unreliable permanent records.

Practices prefer this method because a number system avoids broadcasting a patient's first and last name to the reception area. The number system does not avoid mispronouncing names because names may be mispronounced when the patient presents to the desk or in the exam room. A number system is not more efficient than a registration system because calling a name or a number takes the same amount of time. Sign-in sheets may or may not serve as permanent records of patient activity in a provider's office using an EMR.

5. After seeing Mrs. Simpson, Dr. Stone refers her to a specialist. Which of the following helps make the necessary referral paperwork simple and quick at check-out?

    A. Insurance verification process
    B. Online appointment scheduling
    C. Health maintenance reminders
    D. Customized templates

Customized templates make it simple and quick to add a patient's name to a prewritten referral letter. Insurance verification is required for every office visit. However, it does not make the referral paperwork process simple and quick. An online appointment scheduler allows patients to schedule their appointments online, eliminating telephone calls to the provider. This has no impact on referral paperwork at check-out. Health maintenance reminders are automatic generated messages to the provider that mean a required action is needed in relation to maintaining a patient's health status.

6. An older adult patient seen that day reports his medical history includes "sugar" on both sides of his family. While Karen knows this refers to diabetes mellitus, she also realizes it is important for providers to document precisely in the EHR. Which of the following helps standardize data elements and descriptions of medical terms in the EHR?

    A. **SNOMED-CT**
    B. ICD-10-CM
    C. CPT-4
    D. HCPCS

SNOMED-CT is a medical reference vocabulary that standardizes data elements and terms in EHR systems. ICD-10-CM is a coding classification system that billers, coders, and providers use to document diagnoses. CPT-4 is the coding system providers use to capture provider, diagnostic, and therapeutic services. HCPCS codes capture supplies and non-provider services that cannot be captured with CPT codes.

7. A transport ambulance service the facility partially owns brought in one of the patients that day. The coder was unable to assign a CPT code for the service. Which of the following actions should the coder perform to obtain reimbursement?

    A. Bill the patient directly for the ambulance transport.
    B. Write off the charges because the facility partially owns the ambulance.
    C. Submit a claim form with a HCPCS Level II code.
    D. Assign a CPT code that resembles a nonemergency ambulance transport.

HCPCS Level II codes capture non-provider services. When a patient has insurance, billing the patient directly should be a last resort. The coder should not consider writing off charges when a code assignment is not obvious. Assigning a CPT code that resembles a nonemergency ambulance transport would be coding for something that did not occur, which constitutes fraud.

Quality Documentation at the Patient Bedside

Jordan, the EHR specialist, and Valerie, the nursing shift supervisor, are talking outside a patient's room in the hospital hallway.

"We're looking forward to having all this data available, but a lot of us are nervous about learning a new system," Valerie says.

"Don't be nervous. Our team is here to support you until everyone feels comfortable with the technology. I promise you, in two weeks, you won't know how you lived without computers," Jordan replies.

Jordan and Valerie laugh quietly as Paul, a nurse, comes out of the patient's room.

"Mrs. Eaton is happy to be the first patient to test out the new computer," Paul says.

"Great! Let's get started," Jordan says.

"Sure, I've already taken some vitals," Paul says.

Before entering the room, Jordan looks to the sign on the wall to confirm the patient's name and room number.

Jordan wheels the COW into the patient's room, and Valerie and Paul follow.

"Good morning, Mrs. Eaton. Thank you for allowing us to start the EHR training with you this morning. My name is Jordan Brinks, and I'm with the HIM department. We used to be called medical records, but now with all these computers, we are Health Information Management. I'll be teaching Paul and Valerie how to use this computer to document the care they provide to you and their other patients."

"I find this stuff fascinating, but what's an EHR? I thought you were using a computer?" Mrs. Eaton asks.

"EHR stands for electronic health record. It's your individual health care record. But instead of being papers in a folder, it's on a computer," Paul replies.

"Paul, why don't you get started on the assessment while I get the program up and running," Jordan says.

"Okay, Mrs. Eaton, I'm going to go ahead and do the same things we did yesterday morning. I already got your pulse and respirations so I need your temperature and blood pressure and then ask you some general questions about how you're feeling. It might take a little longer today since I'm entering this information into the computer instead of writing it on my notepad," Paul says.

"You go right ahead, and do whatever you need to do. I'm happy to help!" Mrs. Eaton says.

"Start by logging into the system with your ID and password you set up this morning," Jordan says.

Paul walks over to the COW and enters his username and password using the keyboard. Then, he clicks the mouse to hit enter.

"Now, click on that dropdown menu box to find your patient," Jordan says.

Paul clicks the mouse again.

"Now, find the tab for vital signs," Jordan says.

Paul clicks the mouse once more.

"I'm there! I guess now we need some data," Paul says.

"That's right," Jordan says.

Paul pumps a bottle of alcohol-based sanitizer twice and rubs his hands together.

"Okay, Mrs. Eaton, let's get your vital signs documented so we can leave you alone to watch your stories," Paul says.

Paul gets the blood pressure cuff from the wall and places it on Mrs. Eaton's arm. From the drawers of the COW, he picks up the LED thermometer, sanitary thermometer cover, and stethoscope. He puts the sanitary cover on the thermometer and places it into Mrs. Eaton's mouth. He pumps up the blood pressure cuff and places the stethoscope on the inside of her elbow on that same arm, and listens with the stethoscope as he lets air slowly out of the blood pressure cuff. While he is taking these readings, Jordan and Valerie are talking.

"While we do not recommend that you sign in at the beginning of the shift and stay signed in all day, we do recommend logging into the Super-CHART software right as you begin to do your patient rounds. That way when you get to your patient, you can simply access her chart from the census list and not spend a lot of time logging in and finding where you need to begin," Jordan says.

"Yes, staying logged in all day is a security risk for our patients' private health information and a violation of the HIPAA privacy policy we all signed when we were hired," Valerie says.

"Exactly, so it's important to balance all of that as you figure out how to incorporate this new process into your work routines," Jordan says.

"We have a blood pressure of 117/76," Paul says.

Paul turns to the keyboard and enters in the information.

"Good, Paul, and you can tab over to your next data item so that once you get the reading, all you have to do is enter it," Jordan says.

Jordan swivels the COW so the screen is facing the bed, and Mrs. Eaton can see it as he explains the process to Paul and Valerie.

Mrs. Eaton's thermometer beeps and Paul pulls it out of her mouth. He ejects the plastic covering from the thermometer into the trash can and reads the LED display.

"Temperature is 98.4° F," Paul says as he turns to the keyboard and enters in the data.

Paul turns to look at Valerie.

"I had taken her pulse and respirations before we came in, so can I enter those now, too?" he asks.

"Since it was just a few minutes ago, I think it would be okay, but…" Valerie says.

"We strongly recommend you get into the habit of charting as you perform the testing. This way there's a much lower risk of inaccurate data being logged. Now, once you have entered all the vital signs for your shift, you click here to save the recent data," Jordan says, pointing to the top right of the computer screen.

Paul nods in agreement. After he enters the data, he looks at Jordan and Valerie.

"I need to chart the last time she took her antibiotic. When we talked earlier, she didn't remember what time she took her antibiotic at home yesterday, or even if she took it, so I was going to enter DNR in the nurse's notes, but I'm not sure where to access those from this screen," Paul says.

Valerie looks alarmed.

"That's not the abbreviation we want to use. We have a list of approved abbreviations, and those are the only ones we want to use. Let's let Mrs. Eaton rest for now and move on to our next patient," Valerie says.

"Okay. Thank you, Mrs. Eaton," Paul says.

"Thank you!" she replies.

Valerie heads out of the room, and Jordan and Paul follow, rolling the COW with them. They walk a little way down the hall and stop. Valerie turns to Jordan.

"Can we access the approved abbreviations list and other similar items from this computer?" Valerie asks.

"Yes, you can access all of those things," Jordan replies. "That's part of the benefit of having these computers at the bedside. They make tasks like that so much simpler."

"And safer! DNR means do not resuscitate in case of a code, and that's not what Paul was trying to document, at least I hope not!" Valerie says.

"No, I... uh...," Paul says, looking embarrassed.

"I can come back this afternoon and give all the nurses a quick in-service on where these references are on the computer system. I want to make sure we're all on the same page," Jordan says.

"That's great. Thank you," Valerie says.

"I won't leave until everyone knows this system inside and out. I'll be back at 1 p.m., is that okay?" Jordan asks.

"Perfect. See you then," Valerie replies.

Jordan is talking with Sharon, the HIM director of the hospital.

"How did it go this morning on 9 West?" Sharon asks.

"I think they'll do fine. They're very interested in adopting this as part of their workflow," Jordan says.

"That's good. Sometimes people really push back against change like this. But for now, I need you to quickly run some reports for me, if that's okay," Sharon says.

"Sure, no problem."

"Thanks. I want to run the audit report for the ED admissions on getting patients' advance directives signed and uploaded into the EHR. Please pull that data for this past quarter. I need those statistics to take to the Quality Committee meeting tomorrow morning."

Jordan picks up a notepad from the desk and begins writing reminder notes about the assignments.

"I'll get it done and email it to you before I go to lunch, but that reminds me of something," he says. "This morning one of the nurses wanted to use DNR in his nurse's notes to indicate that the patient did not remember something. We need to make sure the approved abbreviations list is up to date online and maybe even put together an FAQ sheet on where to find these things in the system would help."

"That's a good idea. Why don't you work on that, too, since you'll be out on the floors each week until this system is fully implemented."

"Okay, I will," Jordan says, adding to his notes. "I noticed that some of the nursing staff is so excited about the new computers they forgot to make sure others in the room can't hear the information they are discussing with their patients. This makes me think we need to revisit the privacy and security reminders for everyone."

"Yes, I agree. We don't need another visit from the Department of Health about a privacy investigation!" Sharon replies. "Make sure you include the log-in and log-out policy and why it's really important in the patient care units. Last week, I was up on 3 South and noticed that the COW was sitting in the hall outside a patient's room with someone logged in, but no one standing anywhere near! We're going to have to watch closely until people develop better computer security habits."

"I did mention it to several of the nurses this morning and the supervisor. I'll add that to the training in-service I am putting together," Jordan says, making another note in his notepad.

"That's great. You're doing good work Jordan. This transition from paper to electronic records is never easy," Sharon says.

1. Paul almost entered an incorrect abbreviation into Mrs. Eaton's record. If he had already charted the information, which of the following recommendations should Valerie give him to properly maintain the legal patient record?

   A. "Go in and delete that abbreviation. If someone sees that, we could be sued."
   B. "Add an addendum to the nurse's note to indicate the DNR abbreviation was an error. Then, state Mrs. Eaton did not recall when she last took her medication."
   C. "Put in an IT ticket to get that record reset – that way you can chart it correctly."
   D. "Call the HIM department, and ask someone to append the patient's record, indicating the DNR abbreviation is an error."

2. Before she is discharged, Mrs. Eaton's provider wants to see her blood pressure stabilize. Which of the following EHR tools makes this easy to evaluate?

    A. Clinical templates
    B. Flow sheets
    C. Dropdown menus
    D. Online databases

3. In a compliance review, Jordan notices a radiology technician is regularly accessing multiple records of patients assigned to the obstetrical (OB) unit. This is an issue for which of the following reasons?

    A. The radiology technician must have shared his password with a colleague that works on the OB unit, which is a security violation.
    B. No one should be able to access OB records because they are protected like psychiatric records.
    C. Radiology technicians should only be accessing radiology-specific information.
    D. If an EHR user accesses a system outside his assigned area, it increases the risk of introducing a computer virus and infecting patient records.

4. Mrs. Eaton plans to recuperate from her surgery in another state so she can stay with her daughter. Her daughter's family provider will be serving as her temporary provider while she is recovering. To make sure the family provider meets Mrs. Eaton's postoperative needs, the hospital should send which of the following?

    A. CCD
    B. H and P
    C. Operative report
    D. Discharge summary

5. A dietary technician was on the nursing unit when she noticed a man in a suit without a name badge standing at a COW and typing into the keyboard. She initially thought he was a provider, but when she came out of a patient room, she saw him hurry away as two nurses walked toward the COW. As a hospital employee, it is the dietary technician's duty to perform which of the following actions?

    A. Notify the nursing supervisor about the man.
    B. Call IT to inquire if there was any suspicious activity on the network.
    C. Contact the facility's Privacy Officer.
    D. Notify the hospital security department.

Quality Documentation at the Patient Bedside: Answers

1. Paul almost entered an incorrect abbreviation into Mrs. Eaton's record. If he had already charted the information, which of the following recommendations should Valerie give him to properly maintain the legal patient record?

    A. "Go in and delete that abbreviation. If someone sees that, we could be sued."

    B. "Add an addendum to the nurse's note to indicate the DNR abbreviation was an error. Then, state Mrs. Eaton did not recall when she last took her medication."

    C. "Put in an IT ticket to get that record reset – that way you can chart it correctly."

    D. "Call the HIM department, and ask someone to append the patient's record, indicating the DNR abbreviation is an error."

    When addressing an error in documentation, the clinician should append the progress note with documentation that describes the error and notes the correct data. Entries into the legal medical record should not be deleted. Data in the patient record is not an IT issue. While HIM professionals provide guidance on documentation and the components of the legal health record, they do not document in the patient record.

2. Before she is discharged, Mrs. Eaton's provider wants to see her blood pressure stabilize. Which of the following EHR tools makes this easy to evaluate?

    A. Clinical templates

    B. Flow sheets

    C. Dropdown menus

    D. Online databases

    Flow sheets display continuous data, which is data in a time sequence, such as vital signs, over time. Clinical templates help guide the clinical staff to complete documentation. Dropdown menus are useful for EHR users who want to select specific documentation items. Online databases provide convenient access to reference data, such as the Physician's Desk Reference.

3. In a compliance review, Jordan notices a radiology technician is regularly accessing multiple records of patients assigned to the obstetrical (OB) unit. This is an issue for which of the following reasons?

    A. The radiology technician must have shared his password with a colleague that works on the OB unit, which is a security violation.

    B. No one should be able to access OB records because they are protected like psychiatric records.

    C. Radiology technicians should only be accessing radiology-specific information.

    D. If an EHR user accesses a system outside his assigned area, it increases the risk of introducing a computer virus and infecting patient records.

HIPAA limits access to patient information based on the minimum necessary standard. There is no evidence the radiology technician shared his password. All patient records are private, not only OB and psychiatric records. If an EHR user accesses one area of a system as opposed to another area, it does not increase the risk of introducing viruses.

4. Mrs. Eaton plans to recuperate from her surgery in another state so she can stay with her daughter. Her daughter's family provider will be serving as her temporary provider while she is recovering. To make sure the family provider meets Mrs. Eaton's postoperative needs, the hospital should send which of the following?

    A. CCD

    B. H and P

    C. Operative report

    D. Discharge summary

The hospital should send a CCD because it is the method of choice for sharing pertinent medical information between providers. H and P is a document that is important to the inpatient admission and subsequent care. An operative report summarizes any surgical procedures. A discharge summary provides a recap of the admission and includes any patient instructions.

5. A dietary technician was on the nursing unit when she noticed a man in a suit without a name badge standing at a COW and typing into the keyboard. She initially thought he was a provider, but when she came out of a patient room, she saw him hurry away as two nurses walked toward the COW. As a hospital employee, it is the dietary technician's duty to perform which of the following actions?

    A. Notify the nursing supervisor about the man.
    B. Call IT to inquire if there was any suspicious activity on the network.
    C. Contact the facility's Privacy Officer.
    D. Notify the hospital security department.

Due to strict HIPAA regulations regarding protecting patient information and reporting any breach of information, the dietary technician should notify the facility's Privacy Officer so he can assess the situation and take the appropriate action. While it may make sense to notify the nursing supervisor about the man, according to HIPAA it is not the dietary technician's duty. Suspicious network activity may not be detectable even when there is a privacy or security breach. It may make sense to notify the hospital security department, but according to HIPAA it is not the dietary technician's duty.

>> SUMMARY

This study guide helps to prepare you for the CEHRS exam NHA offers. It breaks your duties and responsibilities as an EHR specialist into five chapters: software applications and equipment, insurance and billing, charting, regulatory compliance, and reporting.

The study guide reviews the reasons facilities must replace paper records with electronic health records. Because patients seek treatment in a variety of settings, providers benefit if they can have access to their patients' information quickly. Electronic records also play an important role in the safety, efficiency, and quality of patient care, and help to reduce the cost of health care. Other benefits of the EHR include faster diagnoses, treatment, and test results; the ability to retrieve information easily; access to decision-making tools for standardization of care; and complete information from all health care professionals.

Chapter 1 was a review on how to use EHR software and applications, a vital skill you need as an EHR specialist. The chapter contained two sections: application operation and practice management. The section on application operation focused on how to use, manage, and acquire data in EHR software, whereas the practice management section focused on providing end-user training and support of EHR software.

Chapter 2 contains information on your role as an EHR specialist in insurance and billing. Chapter 2 also provides an introduction to coding by abstracting diagnoses and procedural descriptions from the patient's medical record, entering those descriptions into the appropriate coding software, and finding codes in the ICD-10-CM/PCS, CPT, and HCPCS coding manuals, whether online or in traditional books.

Charting is one of the most important functions of EHR software for a clinician. This is why Chapter 3 emphasizes the importance of providers entering live data in the EHR at the point of care by dictation, transcription, voice recognition software, scanning, or clinical templates. This chapter also focuses on the data within charts. You must monitor patients' charts to ensure they are accurate, secure, and complete, and categorize patients' health information into a reliable and organized system.

As an EHR specialist, you should be familiar with key parts of HIPAA and HITECH. Chapter 4 explained the importance of following HIPAA and HITECH standards. The HIPAA Security Rule protects the integrity, confidentiality, and availability of electronic PHI. To protect electronic PHI, make sure your facility enforces administrative, physical, and technical safeguards. These safeguards may not fully protect the information, so it is important you have a system and a procedure in place for detecting and reconciling threats.

Chapter 5 described how the reporting function of EHR software can be helpful. You can generate statistical reports for clinical and financial QI measures, aging reports by guarantor or insurance carrier, and financial analysis reports by provider, diagnosis, or procedure. You can use a QI report to gather insight into ways a clinician can perform better or more efficiently, or find a way to cut costs. Chapter 5 also explained how to collect medical care and census data for continuity of care records.

Finally, there was a case studies section, which provides you with three real-world scenarios to test your knowledge in all areas of the study guide.

You represent the future of health care. Remain continuously committed to keeping up with changes in the health care system. Consistently strive for greater awareness of others and how to best serve as a member of the health care team. Use the skills you acquire from this study guide to help yourself and other EHR specialists succeed. You are a valued member of the health care field.

References

Abdelhak, M., Grostick, S., and Hanken, M.A., (Eds). (2011). *Health Information: Management of a Strategic Resource, 4th edition*. St. Louis: Saunders.

Buck, C.J. (2012). *Step-by-Step Medical Coding, 2012 edition*. St. Louis: Saunders.

Casto, A.B., and Layman, E., (Eds.). (2009). *Principles of Healthcare Reimbursement, 2nd edition*. Chicago: AHIMA Press.

Johns, M. L. (2011). Health information management technology: An applied approach, 3rd edition. Chicago: AHIMA Press.

U.S. Department of Health and Human Services (DHHS), (n.d.). Health Information Privacy: A Summary of the HIPAA Security Rule. Retrieved from http://www.hhs.gov/ocr/privacy/hipaa/understanding/srsummary.html.

U.S. Department of Health and Human Services (DHHS), (2003). OCR Privacy Brief: A Summary of the HIPAA Privacy Rule. Retrieved from http://www.hhs.gov/ocr/privacy/hipaa/understanding/summary/privacysummary.pdf.